HELPING ABUSED AND TRAUMATIZED CHILDREN

Helping Abused and Traumatized Children

*Integrating Directive
and Nondirective Approaches*

ELIANA GIL

Foreword by John Briere

THE GUILFORD PRESS
New York   London

© 2006 The Guilford Press
A Division of Guilford Publications, Inc.
72 Spring Street, New York, NY 10012
www.guilford.com

Printed in the United States of America

This book is printed on acid-free paper.

Last digit is print number: 9 8 7 6 5 4 3 2

Library of Congress Cataloging-in-Publication Data

Gil, Eliana.
  Helping abused and traumatized children : integrating directive and nondirective
approaches / Eliana Gil.
    p. ; cm.
  Includes bibliographical references and index.
  ISBN-10: 1-59385-334-3   ISBN-13: 978-1-59385-334-1 (cloth)
  1. Child abuse—Treatment.   2. Play therapy.   I. Title.
  [DNLM: 1. Child Abuse—therapy.   2. Child.   3. Family Therapy—methods.
4. Play Therapy—methods. WS 350.2 G463h 2006]
  RJ507.A29G552 2006
  618.92′891653—dc22

                                                              2006010324

3/17/08

Dr. William Friedrich, you were a man of great humility and integrity. I learned so much from you. Your quiet and powerful leadership has inspired and guided me. I am proud to have known you a little, exchanged ideas with you, and had a few laughs. I feel your absence and revere your substantial legacy.

About the Author

Eliana Gil, PhD, is Director of the Starbright Training Institute for Child and Family Play Therapy and dedicates some of her time to providing intensive courses on assessment and treatment of child abuse. She also works at the Multicultural Clinical Center in Springfield, Virginia, where she is developing The Children's Corner to provide mental health services for young children with a range of problems, including child maltreatment. Dr. Gil has focused her work on helping sexually abused children and families for the past 33 years in California, Maryland, and Virginia. She teaches courses on child maltreatment, play therapy, and family therapy at Virginia Tech and has authored several books. Originally from Ecuador, she is bilingual and bicultural.

Foreword

The last several decades have witnessed a dramatic increase in our knowledge of the impacts of trauma on children and adolescents. We have discovered that child abuse and neglect by parents and other caretakers—as well as victimization by peers and adults in the community—can lead to outcomes ranging from anxiety and depression, insecure parent–child attachments, and posttraumatic stress, to aggression, interpersonal problems, eating disorders, substance abuse, and self-endangering behaviors. In fact, it may not be too much of a leap to suggest that exposure to trauma and emotional neglect is one of the prime causes of nonorganic psychological disturbance in North American children and youth.

At the same time, however, we have increasingly discovered that nothing is as simple as a cursory reading of the literature might suggest. For example, we now know that the extent to which a child or adolescent develops trauma-related symptoms is a complex function of a number of potentially interacting variables. These minimally include (1) *predisposing factors*, such as the child's initial neurobiology; the quality of his or her parental attachments; broader social variables, including the child's relative experience of racial or ethnic discrimination, poverty, and diminished resources; and cultural or subcultural influences on his or her perceptions of self, others, and the nature of adversity; (2) *characteristics of the trauma(s)*, including the type, number, duration, and age of onset of trauma exposure—with multiple, early, and extended experiences of intrafamilial abuse and neglect being among the most pathogenic; and (3) *posttrauma variables*, such as overall level of familial and social support;

the child's capacity for emotional expression and help seeking; relative safety from further violence or maltreatment; and whether appropriate psychological treatment is available.

The implications of these various interacting variables for the young trauma survivor—and for those who would treat him or her—are important. Because every child has, to some extent, a different biology, psychology, perceived family environment, social context, trauma history, and postvictimization experience, each is also likely to have a different symptomatic presentation. One child, with a history of positive attachment relationships in the context of caring and nonabusive child rearing, a benign social environment, and a relatively circumscribed and limited trauma by a nonparental figure, may experience only mild anxiety, transient posttraumatic stress, and/or a limited period of social withdrawal. Another child, raised by disengaged, neglectful, and/or abusive caretakers in the context of poverty and social deprivation, who has been exposed to repetitive traumatic experiences within and outside of the family, may experience severe depression, posttraumatic stress disorder, substance abuse, and episodes of suicidality or aggression.

Obviously, these two scenarios require different intervention strategies, since treatment must address different symptoms, etiologies, social issues, and personality styles in each case. In the first instance, the family system is stable, attuned, and supportive. The therapist may easily involve the parents and other family members in assisting the child, and the treatment plan may be relatively straightforward. Family therapy may be used to augment play, art, or "talk" therapy (depending on the age of the child), during which the child is encouraged to process memories of the traumatic event until they no longer evoke symptomatology. Because the child is not overwhelmed by posttraumatic symptoms and has a history of being able to trust and rely on adults, he or she is likely to engage in treatment without undue hypervigilance, avoidance, or functional impairment. All other things being equal, the immediate prognosis for this child is likely to be good.

Sadly, most therapists who deal with traumatized youth are more likely to see the second scenario: a highly symptomatic child or adolescent in a relatively unsupportive (if not hostile) environment who has learned to deal with trauma either through avoidance or via "acting-out" responses. Further, because he or she has learned that adults can be dangerous, and that emotional attachment is a recipe for potential abandonment, this second child may not easily permit the development of a meaningful therapeutic relationship, let alone fully participate in serial experiences of vulnerability in the context of an authority figure. More than for others, therapy for this child will have to take his or her relational injury into account; the clinician must provide demonstrable safety, relational consistency, and empathic attunement, and may have to be especially patient with the client as his or her triggered trauma responses impinge on the therapeutic process. Further, the multiple targets of treatment in such cases (e.g., years of childhood sexual abuse and/or emotional neglect, and/or multiple peer victimization experiences in a continuously dangerous community environment) will, of necessity, complicate—and often extend—therapy.

Of course, as demonstrated in this book, it is not even that simple. There is no "second scenario," per se. When multiple, interacting predisposing vulnerabilities and complex traumatic events converge in the same child, there is often no single syndromal outcome to diagnose, nor any definitive one-size-fits-all treatment manual to consult. Instead, treatment has to be customized for each child, based on ongoing assessment of his or her specific psychological injuries, capacities, and attachment style. Although all effective treatment is likely to involve a good therapeutic relationship, emotional validation, exposure-based processing of trauma memories, and the reworking of distorted cognitions, the way in which these and other goals are implemented (i.e., their timing, context, intensity, and order of attention) will necessarily vary from child to child. In this regard, neither the "forest" nor "the trees" of therapy can be overlooked: The goal is to both (1) provide rational, components-based treatment that reflects current empirical research and clinical experience, and (2) take into account the child's individual symptoms, needs, vulnerabilities, and personality.

It is within this growing understanding of the complexities of trauma and treatment that Eliana Gil's new book appears. A mindful, pragmatic thinker with many years of experience in working with abused children, Dr. Gil provides the reader with an integrative text on the treatment of traumatized children and adolescents. As is necessary in any modern clinical treatise, this book incorporates a wide range of therapeutic approaches and includes detailed and useful information on the potential interface between empirically validated and expressive treatment techniques. An equally important contribution is the author's "real-world" attention to the lived experience of the traumatized child. Dr. Gil is adept at discerning the many forces and adaptations that influence the traumatized child's ongoing experience and response to therapy, as well as articulating the need for creative, intelligent interventions that call on both technology and, ultimately, humanity.

JOHN BRIERE, PHD
Associate Professor of Psychiatry and Psychology
Keck School of Medicine
University of Southern California

Preface

I worked with Camila throughout her disclosure of sexual abuse by her father, her medical exam, her father's arrest, testimony in court, the father's sentencing, and her parents' ensuing divorce. Through it all she was fiercely loyal to her father, remained intensely hopeful, and resisted feelings of guilt and shame. Eventually the floodgates opened, and with this came healing. In our final session we looked back at all that had occurred, and she sighed deeply. "We've moved a lot of mountains," she said in a whisper. "Thank you." "Thanks for trusting me," I responded, amazed at her ability to describe the hardship of doing therapy and grateful to have been by her side during this reparative process. I have written this book for Camila and hundreds of other children who have shown me they can heal from overwhelming injuries, who have touched my heart, and who have given me great inspiration.

Since I wrote *The Healing Power of Play* in 1984, several significant personal and professional events occurred in my life: I relocated to the East Coast, and I had two opportunities that stimulated and expanded my creative thinking and subsequently my work. First, I enrolled in George Washington University's Art Therapy Program and became a registered art therapist after years and years of wanting to pursue this formal training. This training experience was both personally and professionally enriching for me. In addition, after many years of lecturing nationally and internationally, I became eager to settle down and focus my attention on developing a sexual abuse treatment program—one that would incorporate the many lessons I had learned over years of trial and error. Through serendipity, I found the Inova Kellar Center, a behavioral treatment facility for children and adolescents in Fairfax, Virginia. The center is affiliated with Inova Fairfax Hospital, home of one of the best sexual abuse nurse examiner (SANE) programs in the United States. Inova Kellar Center had received a grant to start a treatment program for sexually abused children, and its directors had begun a national search for a coordinator. I was in their back yard, and luckily we found each other. From the outset, it was clear to me that Inova Kellar's directors had established a one-of-a-kind treatment facility providing a range of high-quality services to children and their families. Their interest in sexual abuse treatment was in keeping with their commitment to respond to gaps in community services. They gave me ample room to develop the Abused Children's Treatment Services (ACTS) program, now entering its eighth year and currently under the capable direction of Sarah Stoudt Briggs. This opportunity to design a treatment program came at a perfect time for me, given my recent immersion in the study of the expressive arts, which complemented my previous work with children.

Throughout my 33 years in the field of prevention and treatment of child abuse, I have learned a lot from my child clients. In particular, I have learned to meet each child as a unique individual whose needs will become apparent as I get to know him or her. There is no agenda on my part except to make children feel comfortable and safe by observing and listening; being emotionally present; and trying to understand their perceptions, feelings, and behaviors. Once this process occurs, I try to respond to their needs in the best way I can. Some children choose to talk; others play and draw; still others read books, write in journals, or watch videotapes. Therapy means different things to different children, and I remain as flexible as I can be.

I am filled with admiration for the resiliency of injured children, as well as for both the complexity and the simplicity with which the healing process unfolds. It is tempting to focus on doing the right thing, using the latest prop, asking the right questions, or giving the most enlightened advice. But often the most critical help I can give is to take advantage of those decisive moments when what I need to do is *get out of the way* and let children do what they need to do to help themselves. The older I've gotten, the easier it has become to trust the process and wait calmly. The anxiety and tensions of my youth have long passed.

I am keenly aware of the current pressures in mental health care to "hurry up"—to keep treatment as brief as possible for the sake of cost containment. I cannot disagree more with this economically driven approach. As I lecture on the topic of treating abused children, I notice a trend in audience members' questions about how to accomplish trauma work in shorter amounts of time. I think that this trend is misguided. We need to hold fast to the notion that psychological injuries take time to heal, and that we need to afford children whatever amount of time it takes for them to achieve a sense of personal safety and control. The length of treatment is not predictable, because each child's experience and response to the experience will be different. We see this difference clearly in recovery time for physical problems. I worry that we promote a dangerous myth in mental health care when we respond to external pressures by designing treatment approaches focused primarily on shorter lengths of stay. This response seems short-sighted, superficial, and potentially dangerous. I believe that trauma work takes time—not careless or vague use of time, and not a predetermined exact amount of time, but structured and goal-focused time.

In the pages that follow I present a treatment model based on my work at the Inova Kellar Center. This model has been developed in the course of my own professional maturation, and it represents an integration of several grounding theories. I present the context of the work in the first part of the book, and illustrate the implementation of these ideas in the second part.

Although I now work at the Multicultural Clinical Center in Springfield, Virginia, I was blessed with an exceptional staff in the ACTS program at Inova Kellar, with whom I engaged in collaborative decision making and constant dialogue about how to improve and continue shaping our services. Many ACTS staff members' ideas are highlighted in this book. I am particularly indebted to Sarah Stoudt Briggs, Silvina Hopkins, Kirsten Lundeberg, and Virginia Huici, as well as to numerous colleagues who have made contributions to my thinking over the years. These have included Kay Washington, Lisa Wright, Holly Warren, Kristy Howlett, Sofia Travela, Henry Stribing, and Wes Smith; I must also thank our stellar interns at ACTS, Michelle Ward, Cindy Matthies, Diana Bermudez, Erin Morgan, Barry Alvarez, Sung Han, Monica Nava, Holly Boink, and Kitty Shepley. Finally, it was my great fortune to work closely with Beth Iddings (and her awesome staff), supervisor of the sexual abuse unit of Child Protective Services in Fairfax, Virginia, as well as with Sue Brown (and her excellent personnel), director of the SANE program at Inova Fairfax Hospital. Our supportive and mutually respectful collaboration allowed us to provide optimal services to the families we served.

The question I am most often asked is this: "How do you keep yourself optimistic or hopeful while you do this work?" My response? It is an ongoing challenge and requires constant evaluation and mindful action. It has been sad for me to witness some of my colleagues change professions over the years, dismantle long-term intimate relationships, develop drinking problems, and experience periods of depression and fatigue.

These have served as reminders that clinicians are vulnerable to the stressors and demands of witnessing and "being with" the painful emotions of others.

I share the information in this book with great humility. I sometimes marvel at the professional respect that I have achieved and the number of people who listen to what I say. It is both a responsibility and an honor that I treat with great care. It is my hope that my ideas serve as springboards to clinical creativity. I deeply appreciate my clients' trust in me, as well as yours. I accept it respectfully.

ELIANA GIL

Contents

PART I

The Context for Clinical Work

1

Basic Principles for Working with Abused and Traumatized Children

The purpose of this book is to emphasize the necessity and applicability of an integrative approach to working with children, especially abused and traumatized ones. This approach recognizes children's linguistic and cognitive limitations and their varied developmental levels, as well as the clinical challenges frequently presented by children's resistance to a therapy process that is often unfamiliar and that they themselves infrequently seek out. In addition, children who are physically or sexually abused (especially the latter) are often genuinely resistant to speaking about their emotional and bodily injuries at all. This is true whether children are abused within or outside their families, but when these injuries occur at the hands of loved and trusted caretakers, the resulting conflicts may completely compromise children's ability and/or willingness to address difficult thoughts and feelings.

My career currently spans 33 years, and during that time I have worked with thousands of abused children (and their families or caretakers), briefly or on a long-term basis. I have grown to value the unique nature of each child, his or her family members, and their recovery process. Because of clients' individuality, I firmly believe that clinicians who remain conversant with multiple theories and approaches will be the most successful at engaging and maintaining children and their families in treatment. Following the description of a comprehensive assessment (see Chapter Two), I summarize treatment goals (Chapter Three). I then encourage an integration of expressive therapies (art, play, and sand, discussed in Chapter Four) designed to engage nonverbal and acutely resistant children, as well as cognitive-behavioral therapy (CBT) for children who are verbal and can participate in this type of therapy (see Chapter Five). I don't see these approaches as exclusive, single modes of therapy, but as complementary and mutually beneficial. Of course, child therapy presumes that children will be assessed and treated within their family, community, and cultural systems. Chapter Six therefore discusses the essential aspect of working systemically with abused children, for whom relationships and interpersonal exchanges can become complex. Work with this population can also involve some special issues, such as posttraumatic play and the presence of dissociative responses in many abused children; these exceptional clinical challenges are addressed in Chapter Seven. The second part of the book offers four clinical case examples to illustrate the possibilities of integrative work for optimal results.

My work is anchored in several basic theories, as well as specific beliefs that have emerged through the practice of meeting abused children and their families—all of whom receive therapy because of similar events in their lives, and yet all of whom are clearly distinctive. These beliefs inform and guide therapeutic work based on clients' needs at different phases of treatment. These beliefs and subsequent approaches are consistently reevaluated and may be emphasized or utilized to a greater or lesser extent, depending on emerging empirical data, ongoing clinical experience, or the fluctuating needs of a child and family. I am most strongly influenced in this stage of my life by trauma theory; the evidence for how children use their instinctive drives to negotiate trauma (with greater or lesser success); the interface of CBT and expressive therapies; my own and others' observations of the remarkable stabilizing effects of resiliency; the overwhelming evidence for the effects of severe and/or chronic stress on children's neurobiology (as well as emerging data on the possibility of reversing some of these effects); and the relevance of contextual/systemic work. Finally, this work requires consistent acknowledgment and processing of countertransferential responses, and this processing is inherently connected to the development and establishment of responsible self-care practices.

TRAUMA THEORY: THE IMPORTANCE OF ASSESSING TRAUMA'S PRESENCE AND IMPACT

The word (and concept) "trauma" has been consumed by popular vernacular to such an extent that it is now often applied to taking exams, getting haircuts, making speeches, traveling, shopping in crowded stores, and other typically mundane events. When the word is used as diffusely as in these examples, it appears that the intent of communication is to describe something as stressful, demanding, or uncomfortable. This excessive and imprecise use of the word "trauma" dilutes its true meaning and confuses its intended message.

In the area of child abuse and neglect, the words "abuse" and "trauma" are frequently used interchangeably, as if they were synonymous. Instead, I believe it is necessary to differentiate these words and subsequent concepts (and use them purposefully), because traumatized individuals may have different therapeutic needs from those of individuals who have experienced acute stress but who do not suffer long-term traumatic impact. To begin with, the *Diagnostic and Statistical Manual of Mental Disorders*, fourth edition, text revision (DSM-IV-TR; American Psychiatric Association, 2000) defines a traumatic event as follows:

> . . . an event that involves actual or threatened death or serious injury, or other threat as to one's physical integrity; or witnessing an event that involves death, injury, or a threat to the physical integrity of another person; or learning about unexpected or violent death, serious harm, or threat of death or injury experienced by a family member or other close associate. (p. 463)

Van der Kolk (1987) notes that the critical issue in defining trauma and its resolution is the *debilitating loss of control* that individuals, especially young children, experience (in other words, he emphasizes the phenomenological aspect). This loss of control has significant consequences:

> . . . if the distress is overwhelming, or when the caregivers themselves are the source of the distress, children are unable to modulate their arousal. This causes a breakdown in their capacity to process, integrate, and categorize what is happening. At the core of traumatic stress is a breakdown in the capacity to regulate internal states. If the distress does not ease, the relevant sensations, affects, and cognitions cannot be associated—they are dissociated into sensory fragments—and as a result, these children cannot comprehend what is happening or devise and execute appropriate plans of action. (van der Kolk, 2005, p. 403)

The effects of traumatic events can often last over long periods of time, waxing and waning. They may be manifested in the symptomatic behaviors associated with posttraumatic stress disorder (PTSD), even if an individual does not meet full criteria for a formal diagnosis of PTSD. In particular, they may be exacerbated with exposure to additional stressors (triggers that remind traumatized persons of the original events).

Among people exposed to traumatic events, there is great variety in the type and level of traumatic experiences and effects, as well as in trauma's short- and long-term management. Terr (1991), for example, distinguishes between single-event traumas (Type I) and chronic traumas (Type II). There are also obvious differences among traumatic events that are "acts of God," such as hurricanes, earthquakes, or floods; random events such as car accidents; acts of terrorism against groups; politically motivated torture; and interpersonal acts of assault and injury between strangers (random rape), familiar people (date rape), and family members (incest). Some recent literature also uses the differential descriptors "simple" and "complex" for types of PTSD. Such is the concern with distinguishing among types of trauma effects in children that van der Kolk (2005) has recently proposed a new term to capture a conceptual departure from contemporary definitions. "Developmental trauma disorder," van der Kolk posits, includes "multiple or chronic exposure to one or more forms of developmentally adverse interpersonal trauma; affective and behavioral dysregulation; persistently altered attributions and expectations; and functional impairment" (2005, p. 404). This volume focuses on "developmentally adverse interpersonal trauma" in van der Kolk's sense—specifically, on such trauma as the result of child abuse (especially child sexual abuse). However, it's critical to note that interpersonal acts of child abuse and neglect occur within a larger context that can include additional stressors, such as drug abuse, domestic violence, or environmental stressors (poverty, social oppression, etc.).

Although child sexual abuse is often highlighted in the literature on child abuse and neglect, all forms of child maltreatment have the potential to be traumatic: physical abuse, sexual abuse, neglect or endangerment, and both active and passive forms of emotional abuse. All of these are dangerous to children's development and survival, and children can suffer consequences from them, whether they are intense but brief or long-lasting and persistent. What allows one person to return to normative functioning, while another has a life beset with grave difficulties, is the subject of great speculation and study (and is likely to generate discussion and research for years to come). However, it is clear at this time that traumatized children are a subset of abused children, and that children's responses to abuse are extremely heterogeneous. As O'Donohue, Fanetti, and Elliott (1998) point out, "although we know child sexual abuse can have clinically significant effects for the child, the exact nature of these effects, whether they cluster together in some syndrome, the extent to which problems emerge immediately or are delayed, and factors that mediate or buffer the effects of abuse are largely unknown" (p. 356). Treatment providers are therefore advised to suspend judgment when they are gauging and assessing the impact of trauma. Some trauma specialists tend to expect a maximum impact in all cases, while others may be more disposed to view traumatic responses as transient and manageable. These expectations and assumptions will influence clinical responses.

Because of the wide variation in their responses, maltreated children must be evaluated carefully, so that their individual (and familial) needs can be identified on a case-by-case basis. For example, one child's history of very severe and chronic abuse may signal greater concerns; however, this child may have personality traits that elicit positive, nurturing responses from important people in his or her environment, and thus the child may have the opportunity to form strong and trusting relationships that can be helpful in the recovery process. Another child with a similar or even a less severe history may elicit negative responses from caretakers and peers, and may therefore have difficulty experiencing intimacy with others; this difficulty may compromise his or her ability to trust others or to achieve emotional connectedness. In other words, some children seem to have internal resources to overcome early hardships, and their prognoses are thus often better than those of children lacking such resources. Abused children may fare differently based on many other factors as well, and I describe several types of such factors below.

In order to further illustrate the need for comprehensive assessments of children with histories of abuse or neglect, it is useful to think of the abuse or neglect itself (i.e., the stressor) as having the potential of causing great harm. Individuals may negotiate the stressor differently—and outcomes may differ greatly—depending on their perceptions of the event, coping strategies, available resources (both internal and external), and

TABLE 1.1. Individual Characteristics That May Influence Whether the Traumatic Impact of a Stressor (Abuse or Neglect) Is High or Low

High traumatic impact	Low traumatic impact
Inability to cope is persistent	Coping develops and grows
Coping strategies are lacking or unsuccessful	Coping strategies succeed
Internal resources are unavailable	Internal resources are available
External resources are unavailable	External resources are available
Expressive ability is lacking	Expression is achieved
Symptoms persist	Symptoms decrease
Helplessness persists	Hopefulness increases
Personal control is lacking	Personal control is restored
Existential crisis cannot be resolved	Existential crisis can be resolved
Trauma cannot be resolved or is negatively resolved	Trauma can be resolved

other characteristics affecting their overall management of the experience (see Table 1.1). These characteristics in turn are greatly affected by age; cognitive abilities; prior stressors and previously established coping strategies; temperamental differences; and qualitative differences in motivation, attitude, and resiliency. Changes in brain chemistry and in the ability to manage and restore brain functioning are also critical mediators of how long-lasting or intense potential trauma impact can be.

As noted above, several different categories of factors have been shown to be associated with low or high traumatic impact. In addition to child-related variables (type of trauma, level and duration of trauma, child's age, previous level of functioning, caretaking support, past trauma history), these include trauma-related variables (type, level, and duration of trauma exposure, exposure to traumatic exposure, number and extent of secondary adversities and stressors); caregiver-related variables (past and current psychopathology, trauma history); caregiver–child relationship variables (relationship quality, perception of child); and contextual variables (socioeconomic status, current life stress, family supports) (Bosquet, 2004, p. 302).

Whatever children's circumstances may be, their ability to negotiate trauma naturally should never be underestimated. It is important to note that no two children are alike, that perceptions of the same traumatic event may be quite different, and that the ability to cope cannot be easily predicted. There are at least two primary drives that can emerge during stressful events; I discuss these next.

TRAUMA NEGOTIATION: CHILDREN'S INSTINCTIVE DRIVES

Children seem to negotiate their emotional injuries by utilizing two basic drives that can guide their behaviors. The first drive is to master what is painful or confusing, restoring a sense of control and mastery; the second drive is to avoid painful emotions, thereby eluding attempts to engage in therapeutic work.

When young children are driven by a desire to master their stressors, their primary approach is to tackle their difficulties head-on. These children make efforts to seek understanding about their situations, and they seek out opportunities to overcome feelings of confusion, helplessness, or despair. "Mastery is, most of all, a physical experience: the feeling of being in charge, calm, and able to engage in focused efforts to accomplish goals" (van der Kolk, 2005, p. 408). Thus, when spurred on by a mastery drive, children may engage in dialogues about their concerns or may utilize play activities to symbolize what is most important to them.

For example, a young boy who had been physically and sexually assaulted came into my office, found a scary monster doll, and used the monster to attack a child doll viciously. The boy then found a superhero doll twice the size of the scary monster doll, and used the superhero to scare and chase away the monster. This boy, who was resistant to speaking about his frightening experience, thus exposed himself symbolically to what he feared (in the form of the scary monster), attacked the child doll in play (identification with his own vulnerability and helplessness), and then found the superhero (police, parent, and/or wizard figure) to chase away the danger. In doing so, he began to acknowledge his sense of vulnerability and fear, and at the same time drew upon resources (the possibility of protection) to help him combat the stressor. His ability to do this in symbolic play afforded him control over the sequence of behavior and the outcome, which inevitably allowed him to feel more immediately empowered. Of course, play behavior such as this is best followed up by coaching with parents and caretakers, so that efforts are made in a child's environment to allow or provide continued experiences with mastery and control.

The second instinctual drive in children who experience abuse is to avoid or suppress what is painful. Children can do this in a variety of ways: They can refuse to think about or talk about the abuse; they can avoid all stimuli reminiscent of the abuse; they can withdraw from interactions with others; and they can refuse to use play materials that remind them of people or things connected with the abuse. Such children may have developed "frozen" reactions that need to be stimulated.

Many young abused children simply state, "When I think about that [the abuse], it makes me feel bad, so I don't think [or talk] about it." This makes perfect sense to me: If there is pain associated with specific thoughts, avoidance of those thoughts (and feelings) is self-protective. However, problems can arise if children develop rigid patterns of avoidance. In these cases, suppression is occurring without any processing of difficult or painful emotions or thoughts. Although suppression (consciously choosing to store such emotions or thoughts in memory) can provide immediate relief for children who have been hurt, it requires sustained efforts to maintain, and will not allow children the understanding and mastery they require to achieve closure, focus on the present, and restore normative functioning. When older children tell me that they don't want to think about the abuse, or want to forget it, I emphasize my agreement with that goal and advise them that the best way to put painful memories in the past is first to acknowledge and understand them. I caution them that trying to avoid painful memories by pushing them away can create a "pressure cooker" effect that allows these memories (and their associated thoughts, feelings, and sensations) to remain powerful. Specifically, memories that are suppressed without any processing can later "explode" unexpectedly like a pressure cooker without its regulator, renewing children's feelings of helplessness and vulnerability (in response to the timing and intensity of the unwanted memories).

It is best to avoid pressuring children into talking about abuse when they don't feel ready to do so. If they feel externally pressured, their responses will either be measured and superficial (intended to appease) or angry and resistant (intended to keep others at a distance, and perhaps increasing their wishes for avoidance). When children seem to shut down or actively resist any discussion or processing of painful memories, they will literally be unable to integrate ideas that can be of true help, but may be able to memorize or repeat statements without true meaning or understanding. I believe that children deserve an opportunity to achieve mastery at their own therapeutic pace. Although it is important not to collude with full denial and avoidance, it is equally important to allow children ample room to unfold their stories (verbally or nonverbally) at their own speed and through various types of communication (behavior, play, or verbal and nonverbal language).

Children may utilize other methods besides overt avoidance to suppress the memory of a traumatic event. My very best friend and her two children were in a serious car accident several years ago. The older child was thrown from the car and sustained severe physical injury, while the younger child escaped the accident with barely a scratch. I remember talking with the younger child soon afterward, and he repeated "the story" of the accident in a detailed, energized, rapid way. He did this for weeks on end. However, his affect decreased when he told the story, and he appeared unconnected to the factual events—as if he was telling a story from a film he had watched, or as if it had happened to someone else, not himself or his family. It took a very long while for this child to integrate the experience. That is, he slowly developed the capacity to recall the event when he wanted; to organize the sequence and develop a narration; to feel his feelings at the time he was describing events; to express his emotions as well as his actions; and, finally, not to be overwhelmed by what he felt while thinking about or verbalizing events of the accident. His rapid, repetitive, energized, literal descriptions (which lasted for almost 3 weeks after the accident) was a different way of avoiding what had overwhelmed him, as well as an obstacle to his integration and acceptance of the accident. During this period, his memories of the accident remained disorganized and compartmentalized (i.e., feelings were separate from visual details), in order to protect him from feelings of helplessness and survival guilt.

Yet another example of avoidance was provided by 10-year-old Hayden, who had been sexually abused by a trusted male adult (a youth minister) and had never found it possible to tell anyone. At the same time, due to his age and stage of development, he would spend countless days and nights thinking about the abuse. He blamed himself for not fighting back, for not running away, for not telling his parents, for getting erections when he was fondled, and for touching himself in the dark of his room. He began repeating the abusive behavior with his 4-year-old brother, Jaime. He would plan times to isolate Jaime; he would mastur-bate him; he would stick his finger in his anus; and he would tell Jaime not to tell, "or else." Jaime told his mother after the second occurrence. Hayden then denied doing it, hit his brother in front of his mother, and had a "meltdown," retreating into his room for hours behind a locked door.

The parents discussed the situation, noted Hayden's recent moodi-ness and self-isolation, and decided to bring him to therapy for an assess-ment. Hayden held to his story that his brother was lying, and that what Jaime had said was "gross!" Noting his resistance, I gave him time and space. Eventually, when Hayden made a self-portrait, he included weap-ons "because bad guys are everywhere." This led to his disclosure about a bad guy named Scott who used to be in his church group. Hayden was unable to tolerate the anxiety and confusion generated by Scott's abusive behavior in the context of a special relationship and a religious setting. He felt that he himself was doing something wrong, and he suppressed his thoughts and feelings as well as he could. However, unable to process these stressful thoughts and feelings, and lacking the ability to protect himself or rely on his external supports (his parents), Hayden began to act out what he could not withstand. Hayden had not consciously chosen to repeat the abusive behavior with his brother, and much later into treat-ment, he had an extraordinary flash of insight: "I was trying to tell some-body what was going on when I hurt Jaime." He added, "I didn't mean to hurt him or make him feel bad." Later still, he made a heartfelt apology to Jaime, spontaneously thanking him for telling their parents about his abuse. Hayden's situation demonstrates several psychological constructs: suppression, repetition compulsion, and communication through behav-ior or acting out what cannot be spoken. Difficult thoughts and emotions can therefore be consciously suppressed by older children; however, since those thoughts and emotions have not been understood or worked through, they tend to come forward behaviorally, seeking expression through actions rather than words.

The two drives and defenses of mastery and avoidance can appear separately or together, and can often appear alternately during or be-tween therapy sessions. There are also several variables that can influence which drive becomes a more or less significant mode of functioning. Because children may enter therapy with a primary drive (toward mastery or avoidance), I find it necessary to accommodate my approach to them, rather than the other way around. So in answer to the question "What kind of child therapist are you?" or "What kind of child therapy works best with this population?" my response is that I adjust my approach to each child client. In some ways, this is much more challenging than approaching all children in a similar fashion or assuming that specific client responses will be either absent or present.

THE INTERFACE OF EXPRESSIVE
AND COGNITIVE-BEHAVIORAL THERAPIES

Expressive Therapies

The assumption underlying verbal therapy is often stated as "Talking to someone makes you feel better." I've always found this statement somewhat presumptuous, because talking about problems can sometimes make clients feel worse, more confused, more restless—in essence, more agitated. Talking can also make a problem seem more real, more compelling, and more serious than before, precisely because it is put into words and spoken to another. In addition, there are some troublesome cross-cultural issues about "speaking." Most importantly, people from certain cultures can feel more uncomfortable once they reveal a secret concern (especially regarding family members). After disclosure, they may feel disloyal for mentioning the problem, or they may have to negotiate how to understand the listener's reactions to what is said. A more general concern is that at times, people of all cultures may experience a sense of loss and control when they reveal secrets or discuss private worries and concerns. They may feel tricked, overexposed, resentful, and frightened, as if they've lost control of something indescribable. They may also experience a sense of generic loss or grief once their private thoughts are shared with others.

Of course, talking can also be a great relief, particularly if clients believe that the world will crumble around them if they verbalize something and discover that they are still standing after making their secrets known. Some children feel empowered by speaking, begin to modulate their vocal tones and pitches, and seem to experience a sense of liberation through speaking; at times, they may raise their voices and endow them with more emotion.

At its most basic, verbal communication is the externalization of a problem in words. The ability to use verbal communication is predicated on chronological age, brain development, linguistic abilities, and encouragement either to speak or to "hold your tongue." Cultural differences in parenting may contribute to children's utilization of a primary communication style; that is, parents may either encourage or discourage speaking about personal subjects. Children's temperament and personality traits also determine their primary communication styles. I recently worked with a young child who was encouraged (almost pressured) to speak more both at home and at school, and yet she resisted this primary mode of communication, opting instead for expressive and nonverbal communication. This might change, depending on age, confidence, and future experiences.

Expressive communication is much broader than language; it is the infant's primary mode of contact with the world. Infants and toddlers communicate much sooner than language is available to them. Sign language is ample and valuable. Verbal language is a much more complex form of communication, since it assumes that the speaker and the listener are attributing the same meanings to words, and that the listener is catching all the contradictory nuances or assertions provided by nonverbal communication, tone and pitch, and idiosyncratic use of language.

As a child and family therapist, I learned early on that I needed to enlarge my repertoire of communication and ways of making contact if I was going to be able to work with young children. Expressive therapies allow for broad or narrow, simple or complex, conscious or unconscious, processed or unprocessed externalizations—giving us a glimpse of what's on a child's mind on any given hour of any given day.

In work with children, it is useful to stay within the metaphors or symbols that they generate themselves, without making efforts to move into more reality-based interpretations immediately. For example, I asked an 8-year-old boy to "draw a picture of yourself." He drew a tree, a big rock, and a little squirrel behind the rock (he put the squirrel's tail coming out of the side of the rock and then noted, "The squirrel is behind the rock"). There were many possible ways to approach this child after this drawing. Notice how the following questions or statements might elicit different responses in the child:

"Why is the squirrel hiding behind the rock?" (Demands an answer.)
"That squirrel must be feeling very scared." (Suggests an emotion the
    child might not feel ready to acknowledge.)
"Oh, I can see by your drawing that you're feeling really uncomfort-
    able and shy about being here." (Tells the child how he feels, which
    might offer him a reason to contradict, defend, or feel exposed and
    uncomfortable.)

All of the interpretations guiding these questions and statements would be fair to make, and some clinicians would do so with ease. However, these different interpretations, when shared directly with the child, would move away from the metaphor that the child had provided and abruptly force him to address the clinician's responses. Interpretations may also cause children to withdraw. In the example above, it was likely that the rock was serving as a barrier, which the child probably required at this moment. Commenting directly might make the child feel the need to protect himself even more strongly.

Notice how the following statements or questions would be likely to elicit a different response (it helps if you put yourself in the shoes of the 8-year-old boy who made the drawing):

"What's it like for the squirrel to be behind the rock?"
"How does the squirrel like it that the tree is so nearby?"
"What does the squirrel do with his free time?"
"How long has that rock been in front of the squirrel?"
"When the squirrel peeks out from behind the rock, what does he see?"

Notice that these are not "why" questions, and that they are formulated to express interest in the metaphor created by the child. Although the interpretation of the drawing might be surmised, it would be more fruitful to pursue the expansion of the metaphor to learn more about the child. The worst-case scenario would be losing this child who was available for emotional contact because a clinician felt the need to rush or push ahead without special attention to what the child's metaphors suggested about him.

In work with children, the value of expressive therapies (play, art, and sand therapies in particular) cannot be overemphasized. Although most professionals who work with children have some toys and art materials in their rooms, not all professionals have sought specialized training in order to use expressive therapies to their full potential. The literature on this field has flourished in recent years (see Chapter Four) and is described more completely throughout this book. Simply put, however, expressive therapies allow and encourage opportunities that greatly enhance therapeutic perspectives, especially in work with abused and neglected children. The bottom line is that through expressive therapies (symbols, play, art images, storytelling, dance, music), children can find alternative forms of depicting and regulating their inner worlds. In play therapy (toys, miniatures), children can identify with objects or symbols, project their thoughts and feelings onto those symbols or objects, and then process (or work through) difficult, painful, or conflictual material in a protected and safe way that respects defensive mechanisms and pacing. Sometimes the working through is on the level of unconscious material, using symbols or metaphors. At other times, the working through is cognitive and rational.

Cognitive-Behavioral Therapy (CBT)

Since the early 1990s, the practice of CBT specifically with sexually abused children has been well studied, and the available research strongly suggests that this approach is efficient and valuable for children who are old enough and have sufficient verbal abilities to make use of it (see Chapter Five). The CBT approach targets potential behavioral problems that can develop as a result of cognitive errors' negative effects on emotions—that is, problems involving both behavioral and affective dysregulation. CBT seems to offer relief and guidance to young children who experience sexual abuse and may be confounded by experiences that overwhelm their abilities to perceive the situation accurately, negotiate their emotions, or access appropriate behavioral responses. Both expressive and CBT approaches can be useful to abused children, and clinicians need to decide which (or what combination) of these to use with children on a case-by-case basis, with specific consideration to their individual needs.

Finally, I reiterate that developing a treatment plan is always a unique challenge and will vary greatly, depending on each child's unique personality, temperament, interests, talents, gender, culture, age, and developmental stage. Deciding how to use the different approaches becomes the "art" of therapy. Each child presents a new "canvas," and the content and process of therapy will take form as the therapeutic relationship builds and mutual understanding deepens.

OTHER ISSUES INFORMING TREATMENT

Focus on Resiliency

As my earlier comments on the better prognosis for children with positive personality traits and other internal resources indicate, I have been consistently impressed by the role of resiliency (Klimes-Dougan & Kendziora, 2000) and innate human motivators (such as survival instinct) that can protect children from the effects of otherwise powerful stressors. Traumatized individuals are not inevitably doomed to succumb to the stressors in their lives; with varying degrees of therapeutic support (depending on their circumstances and needs), they can manage, endure, overcome, or triumph over these stressors. Rigid therapy agendas or clinical biases, however, can limit or overwhelm child clients. The most realistic clinical approach is therefore one that includes a structured, purposeful, and comprehensive assessment (discussed in Chapter Two).

The Role of Neurobiology

Recent findings consistently emphasize the need for an understanding of neurobiology in any attempt to determine the impact of severe and/or chronic stressors on young children. Specifically, early stress in the form of childhood maltreatment "produces a cascade of neurobiological events that have the potential to cause enduring changes in brain development" (Teicher et al., 2003, p. 33). More and more data reveal without a doubt that maltreatment in childhood can have enduring negative effects on a child's brain development and functioning (Teicher, 2002). According to Stien and Kendall (2004), "Experiences in childhood influence brain growth through a process called gene transcription, which affects how genes are activated" (p. 6). The specific effects of chronic stress on the brain that have been identified thus far include diminished development of the left hemisphere in general and the left hippocampus in particular; decreased right–left cortical integration; an increased incidence of electro-encephalographic (EEG) abnormalities; and diminished size of the corpus callosum. The reduction in the corpus callosum seems most important, because of this structure's critical role in connecting the two hemispheres of the brain (Teichert, 2004).

Teicher et al. (2003), reviewing these stress-induced effects, state:

> We postulate . . . instead that these alterations in neurodevelopment represent an adaptive, alternative developmental pathway. Stress-induced developmental modifications, triggered by the nature of experience during critical, sensitive stages, are designed to allow the individual to adapt to high levels of life-long stress or deprivation that may be signaled by early stressful experience. If an individual is born into a malevolent and stress-filled world, the manifestations of early stressful experience on later development may serve an adaptive purpose, enabling the individual to mobilize intense fight–flight responses or react aggressively to challenge. On the other hand, these alterations are not optimal for survival and reproductive success in a more benign environment. (p. 39)

Van der Kolk emphasizes that "many problems of traumatized children can be understood as efforts to minimize objective threat and to regulate their emotional distress" (2005, p. 403). He goes on to state that when children have been living in unpredictable environments, they "may experience difficulty developing object constancy and inner representations of their own inner world or surroundings. . . . Without internal maps to guide them, they act instead of plan and show their wishes in their behaviors, rather than discussing what they want" (p. 405).

Since typical brain development occurs in a gradual and progressive manner, abuse in the early years of life can interrupt, alter, or overtax internal resources in many different ways, causing many short- and long-term challenges for children. This important topic, still in preliminary stages of understanding, has been eloquently articulated in an influential text by Daniel Siegel, *The Developing Mind* (1999). Siegel synthesizes concepts and findings from the disciplines of attachment theory, child development, communication, complex systems, emotion, evolution, information processing, memory, narrative, and neurobiology. In doing so, he gives us access to profound interacting variables that allows us a deeper understanding of the potential impact of child abuse on mind, spirit, and body, as well as implications for treatments that might enhance and strengthen the injured person.

However, in spite of what appear to be very gloomy data, current science is becoming more optimistic about the plasticity of the brain and the possibility of some recovery from trauma-induced brain damage. This optimism has stemmed from further thinking about potential reconditioning of brain development—and, in particular, from the beginnings of research on ways to stimulate growth in areas of the brain that might be underdeveloped after exposure to severe stressors. According to Stien and Kendall (2004), "positive experiences (e.g., nurturing from a parent) can activate genes, creating new proteins that can, for example, strengthen healthy neural connections and promote learning" (p. 6).

Brain science can be quite useful in suggesting aspects of treatment with the potential to be helpful in the process of neurobiological restoration. Stien and Kendall (2004), for example, have proposed an "interactive treatment model" based on the principle that environment can change (and rechange) brain circuitry. They state: "On the one hand, how our brain functions determines how we perceive, think, and behave. On the other hand, by changing our thinking and behavior, the organization and functioning of our brain can be retooled" (Stien & Kendall, 2004, p. 12). The interactive treatment model and other implications of brain science for clinical work are explored further in Chapter Three.

The Necessity of Contextual/Systemic Work

No child exists in a vacuum. Childhood is a time for identity formation, establishment of interactional patterns, and maturation in many dimensions. Most importantly, it is a time when children grow and develop through exposure to parental nurturing, protection, guidance, and the formation of adaptive mechanisms and expanded coping repertoires.

Children's relationships to adult caretakers, peers, and educators are pivotal to their continued growth. When we work with children, we need to understand the social and family contexts in which they operate, so that we can assist in whatever ways are necessary. I am committed to working in the best interests of children, which means that I am constantly striving to ensure that children are situated in nurturing, empathic, and safe environments. Many of our child clients are moving through a foster care system in which their placements are not always stable. Although the intent of foster care is to provide children with necessary temporary caretaking in a protective home, many children experience years of multiple placements with varying degrees of stability, contentment, or conflict. In addition, many decisions that are made for children may be perceived by them as nonsensical, confusing, or punitive. Children who are removed from their families may not understand the separation easily or well. They may remain worried about their families, and they may experience significant feelings of loss. Their caretakers may or may not have profound understanding and superb skills to work with their foster children; indeed, in some unfortunate cases, caretakers and children may be uniquely mismatched.

When parents are separated from their children, they may or may not receive helpful services, and thus family reunification may be challenging at best. Parents may feel more or less comfortable providing safe and stable care. In some cases, children are re-placed in homes where virtually no changes have occurred and where little progress has been made in building healthier, more functional parenting approaches. Reunification services must be provided with a clear understanding that disruptions in attachment, transitions, losses, environmental changes, and the initiation and termination of caretaking relationships between children and parental figures will inevitably produce stressors for children and their families.

Clinicians must remain involved with the inherent contextual and systemic issues that abused children bring into treatment. This often means that when working with this population, clinicians must broaden their roles beyond the boundaries of traditional mental healthcare (see Chapter Six).

Monitoring Countertransference and Pursuing Proactive Self-Care

Working with abused and traumatized children and their parents can evoke strong countertransferential responses in mental health professionals. These may become apparent through somatic problems (headaches, nightmares); emotional distress (anxiety, fear, hyperarousal, or depression); social problems (withdrawal from normative social experiences, withdrawal from social contact); difficulties with interpersonal or intimate relationships; sudden inability or unwillingness to continue working (burnout, stressful work relationships); and a host of other concerns (eating disorders, intrusive flashbacks, emotionality): This problem, known as "vicarious traumatization," is now widely understood and discussed (Osofsky, 2004a; Nader, 1994; McCann & Pearlman, 1990). It is considered an important topic for supervision and consultation among mental health professionals in general, and among those clinicians who are routinely exposed to traumatic material in particular.

Clearly, it is critical for clinicians to be constantly alert for the possible presence of countertransference and subsequent effects. When such effects are detected, it is imperative to design action plans designed to prevent long-term negative impact and maximize full involvement with the provision of mental health services. Immediate crisis intervention is required when therapists operate in polar states of hyperarousal or numbness; feel unable to be emotionally present, engaged, objective, and interested in clients' problems; or suffer from personal emotional debilitation. It is therefore necessary to monitor and address personal issues routinely and thoroughly, in order to maximize professional integrity and client safety. In full recognition of the curative powers of play therapy, a colleague and I (Gil & Rubin, 2005) have recently suggested utilizing play therapy techniques to assist clinicians in processing countertransferential responses.

In summary, my message in this chapter (and in this book as a whole) is that working with abused children requires an integrated approach that is flexible and responsive to clients' unique needs. Mental health professionals who pursue this approach must remain conversant with a variety of theories and approaches (both evidence-based and clinically sound), and have the ability to shift perspectives in order to maximize therapy opportunities for their clients. Working with child maltreatment of any type is inimitably challenging, but superbly rewarding. Suspending assumptions, expectations, and firm agendas, as well as monitoring countertransference and maintaining adequate self-care, will result in greater opportunities to be of help to families and children in crisis.

2

Guidelines for
Integrated Assessment

THE MULTIDISCIPLINARY FRAMEWORK
FOR ASSESSMENT AND TREATMENT

The assessment and treatment of abused and traumatized children present unique challenges. Traditional psychotherapy boundaries are stretched by the necessity for multidisciplinary work and extensive case management; the focus on child safety; the expansion of clinical roles to include advocacy and interfacing with judicial systems; and special attention to the prevention of burnout and vicarious traumatization.

Identification and/or disclosures of child physical abuse, sexual abuse, or neglect set into motion a multilayered response that usually includes investigatory personnel (police officers and/or representatives of the local child protective services [CPS] or department of family services [DFS]); medical exams; referral to mental health services (and crime victim services); arrests of adults who have committed criminal behaviors; removal of children from their homes (and subsequent maintenance in foster care, with permanency planning as a goal); and a variety of court hearings and procedures, in which children may or may not testify. In addition, children and their families may interact with lawyers (including attorneys acting as *guardians ad litem* for children) and with court-appointed special advocates, who assist children throughout court procedures and make recommendations to the court. Within the standard course of a family's interaction with the multiple agencies and subagencies involved in child abuse cases (for the purposes of assessment, treatment, and advocacy), agency personnel may change. For example, in the CPS there are social workers who conduct initial investigations and then others who do case management subsequent to the initial investigations. However, if a child or children are removed from a family home, the family's case is transferred to another social worker within the same agency (DFS) but within a different department (foster care and adoption), who will oversee the placement of the child(ren) in foster care, as well as the reunification process if one is undertaken. If a decision is made to terminate parental rights, a judicial process occurs, and the child or children are released to an adoption worker in order to identify prospective adoptive families.

Clinical services are best provided within a multidisciplinary framework in which a team approach is utilized. It is relevant and helpful to the success of assessment and long-term treatment to establish and maintain a positive working relationship with agency personnel involved in all aspects of service delivery to families. Mental health services are a critical part of the overall response to families in which child abuse or neglect occurs, and we therapists must make efforts to provide or cooperate with coordinated case management in order to help families and their children most effectively. Mental health professionals may feel uncomfortable or awkward taking the lead in case management, and doing so may defy clinicians' beliefs that families will respond with resistance to their collaboration with other agencies. Many clinicians voice a number of concerns in this regard—mainly that the clients' confidentiality may be breached; that clinicians may find their roles compromised; or that the demands for case management and possible court work may be time-consuming, stressful, or literally impossible to provide due to financial constraints. In particular, working primarily with child sexual abuse will require that these issues be resolved in favor of developing creative strategies for increased interaction with outside professionals. For example, it is not unusual for therapists working with such cases to call together professional meetings, arrange conference calls, attend review meetings with family members, discuss legal issues (including testimony) with attorneys, and otherwise maintain a high level of involvement in order to best serve their clients.

Those who specialize in childhood trauma, especially cases of interpersonal abuse, must provide mental health services while maintaining a focus on safety issues and the best interests of children. They must often render opinions about children's placements, the psychological impact of children's testifying in court, the physical and emotional safety of children's environments, and families' ability and willingness to decrease high-risk factors for children (such as drug abuse, domestic violence, etc.).

Mental health services are often provided in tandem with legal services, and it is critical to remain well informed about the ongoing status of legal procedures and time frames in order to avoid compromising a child's best interests in judicial procedures. For example, if child clients are scheduled to testify in a criminal trial, we will not show the child videotapes of child sexual abuse at that particular time.[1] We remain conscientious about the inherent adversarial issues in court proceedings, and we avoid activities that could be considered suggestive or that could compromise the child's credibility. When we refer children to group therapy, we try to make sure that the legal procedures (if any) have already occurred, in order to prevent the children's legal cases from being challenged by defense attorneys who may seek to "muddy the waters" with accusations that group contamination is occurring (i.e., that the group members are emulating one another and getting confused about the facts of their own cases). Clinicians working in child sexual abuse cases are advised to keep abreast of areas of controversy and relevance in the field, either by reading, by attendance at conferences, coursework (Conte, 2002) and by membership in professional organizations (e.g., the American Professional Society on the Abuse of Children).

Those professionals who seek to be of service in child sexual abuse cases must also be well versed in child and family therapy specific to this area of study (Sheinberg & Fraenkel, 2001; Maddock & Larson, 1995; Trepper & Barrett, 1989) and must develop a variety of strategies to successfully engage and assist younger and older children, as well as parents or other caregivers with varying levels of cooperation. Clinicians are advised to maintain child-friendly atmospheres and to stay conscientious about systemic and contextual concerns—that is, to provide services to the immediate and extended family when appropriate and possible, as well as to interact with larger systems such as schools, day care programs, and other health services. Comprehensive and individualized assessment plans set the stage for successful provision of services to all parties.

THE PROCESS OF EXTENDED DEVELOPMENTAL ASSESSMENT

A measured, comprehensive, and sensitive assessment both informs and initiates treatment. Because we work with children in a broad age range

---

[1] As noted in the Preface, I now work at the Multicultural Clinical Center in Springfield, Virginia. However, because the treatment model described in this book was crystallized during my work at the Abused Children's Treatment Services (ACTS) program at the Inova Kellar Center in Fairfax, Virginia, I refer in this book to my ACTS colleagues and myself as "we," and to our work at the ACTS program in the present tense.

(1½–18 years old), we pay particular attention to developmental functioning. In addition, we strive to provide services that are gender- and culture-sensitive (Friedrich, 1990; Gil & Drewes, 2005).

Most clinicians working with this population will encounter myriad external pressures to assess children quickly. Funding sources often demand speedy evaluations and even speedier treatment. Scheduled court dates may also seem to necessitate rapid interventions. Finally, the acuteness of children's symptoms may provoke the need to render prompt diagnoses in order to obtain immediate assistance. We make efforts to educate referring sources about the need and desirability of a comprehensive approach that allows children the time required to develop a safe and trusting relationship with members of the clinical staff.

We have found it best to work in a manner that gives us the best chances of understanding each child and family's unique situation. What we call our process of "extended developmental assessment" includes an intake meeting with parents or caretakers, obtaining historical data and baseline behavioral concerns, and conducting between 10 and 12 individual sessions with children and/or other family members. Obviously, this assessment process will be abandoned in favor of crisis intervention in cases of acute assault such as a single violent rape or gang rape, which will require immediate, direct, and structured responses (Foa & Rothbaum, 1998). These clients (and other especially distressed clients) may then be referred for psychiatric evaluations for hospitalization or medication, and may require participation in structured residential programs (for stabilization purposes) prior to outpatient care.

Many of the cases discussed in this book relate to chronic incest situations within established familial relationships. Extrafamilial abuse may often (though not always) be less complex than intrafamilial abuse, particularly when the persons who have abused children are strangers. In these cases, for the most part, children may perceive that the hurtful events occurred outside their homes and that they can turn more easily to their parents or caretakers for needed support and restoration of security. On occasion, however, parents are not reliable resources, especially at the disclosure stage; they may find the abuse incredible, or they may blame their children for not telling sooner, for not stopping the abuse, or for somehow sharing responsibility for the situation. In addition, parents' guilt for failing to protect their children can temporarily interfere with their ability to be empathic or supportive. Children may be surprised to hear that their parents didn't know about the abuse, may feel afraid that they have done something wrong, may feel anxious about what happens to the abusers, and may harbor resentment or anger against parents who failed to protect them from abuse. Of course, sometimes the complexities of extrafamilial abuse can rival the complexities of incest—for example, when children are manipulated by very charismatic and otherwise caring adults or older children, in the context of long-term interactions in which relationships are established and developed over time (see the case example of Gene, below).

Intake Session

The intake session routinely lasts 1 hour, and typically one or both birth parents attend the interview without the child. Legal guardians may also attend the intake session, including social workers, family members, or foster parents. In this session, written materials (including a developmental and social history form) are completed by parents, reviewed with clinicians, and clarified or expanded if necessary.

Parents or caretakers are then asked to describe the child's allegations; method of disclosure and adult responses; current or past involvement with professionals; and the child's current status and living situation. We also gather data about parental or caretaker concerns and observations. We obtain signed consent forms to speak to relevant professionals, such as social services or school personnel. We then explain our extended developmental assessment and distinguish between such an assessment and a forensic evaluation. It is possible that the intake session may result in referrals to higher levels of care or in a mutual agreement that another clinical service may be more appropriate.

Lastly, parents or caretakers are asked to fill out a variety of paper-and-pencil questionnaires, in addition to federally required privacy forms (mandated by the Health Insurance Portability and Accountability Act, or HIPAA) and a psychosocial and developmental history. These questionnaires include the Child Behavior Checklist (CBCL; see www.aseba.org; separate forms are now available for children ages 1½–5 and 6–18) and the Child Sexual Behavior Inventory (CSBI; Friedrich, 1997). This information provides clinicians with important adults' perceptions of the child's overall functioning, problem areas, social environment, academic progress, and strengths. It also offers a baseline for future assessments of the child's of progress (as reported on these same forms).

The intake session routinely includes some degree of parental coaching, because parents and caretakers have myriad reactions to their children's disclosures or behaviors. The most common questions and worries surround the issue of bringing up the issue of abuse—whether it's better for children if parents "forget" about the abuse or don't mention it at all, or what specifically they should say or do if their children bring up the topic. Cultural differences will greatly influence individuals' comfort with therapy, willingness to discuss family problems with outsiders, views regarding treatment, and level of motivation to avoid or address what has occurred in the family. Children's disclosures can also trigger memories of parents' histories of similar past events, which can add further to the emotional distress they may experience and may even require their parallel abuse-specific treatment.

If the person who abused a child is a trusted family friend or relative, parents must also decide what they will say to other family members. In these circumstances, the restoration of the victimized child's and family's control and power is the overriding goal. Parents need to become well informed about how to respond to their children (both the abused child and any siblings), and they need to make decisions about how to differentiate between privacy and secrecy within their extended families, with special attention to not placing additional pressure on themselves or their children. Cases of sibling incest seem to generate the most acute family distress, in that parents must sort out their thoughts/feelings regarding the child or adolescent who performed the sexual abuse, as well as their thoughts/feelings regarding the abused child. Competing emotions regarding protection and retaliation can be intense and spark overwhelming emotions in family members.

Parents typically struggle with their own emotions of guilt, shame, anger, and despair, which can feel initially overwhelming. They can develop vicarious traumatization and develop symptoms of PTSD (emotionality, intrusive thoughts, flashbacks, hypervigilance, etc.); they may also be susceptible to intense feelings of anger and retaliation (these are most typical in fathers, who often speak of wanting to kill the persons who have hurt their children). In cases of incest, the parents who have not abused (usually mothers) experience feelings of shock, confusion, despair, initial disbelief, and acute distress. Although coaching can be viewed as helpful, some parents may require additional services to assist them in periods of intense crisis. These may include individual or group therapy, as well as in-home services, financial and housing assistance, and so forth.

This coaching is provided during the intake session and then before and after children's sessions, through weekly appointments when needed, or through liberal phone contact as necessary for effective management of the case.

Assessment Sessions with Child Clients: Format, Assumptions, and Goals

Even the youngest abused children (especially sexually abused children) can be vulnerable to the reactions of parents and caretakers. Parental expressions of anger, sadness, or worry can be magnified in children's minds and often misunderstood. Children may come to believe that it's best to avoid the subject in order to protect parents from feeling pain.

Thus meeting with sexually abused children separately from their parents or caretakers is usually good practice for at least part of the time. When children become comfortable with their therapists, they will be more likely to ask questions, make statements, and generally show their perceptions, thoughts, and feelings through a series of verbal and nonverbal activities. Children typically attend once-weekly sessions, although clinicians may suggest more or less frequent sessions, depending on their needs.

Our model of extended developmental assessment allows clinicians to develop age- and gender-appropriate recommendations based on an understanding of each child's general functioning. Two basic assumptions guide the assessment process. First, most sexually abused children who are referred for our services have been interviewed by at least two professionals prior to coming to ACTS; therefore, children are often hesitant to answer further questions or volunteer information about alleged or confirmed sexual abuse. In addition, children who are abused have unique and widely varying responses to their experiences, including acute or chronic symptoms, emotional or behavioral difficulties, relational problems, issues with aggression, or generalized fear and anxiety. In other words, their functioning may be slightly, moderately, or severely impaired.

When clinicians conduct assessments or evaluations of abused children and their family members, generic guidelines regarding child interviews (including interviewing preschool children; Hewitt, 1999), structured clinical interviews and instruments, and psychological evaluations serve as a necessary foundation (Friedrich, 2002b; Hughes & Baker, 1991; Samuels & Sikorsky, 1990; Greenspan, 1981). It is also extremely important for therapists to utilize their intuitive abilities as well as their countertransferential responses (Gil & Rubin, 2005). The extended developmental assessment follows a formal and established course at first. In the early phase (i.e., the first three or four sessions), clinicians focus exclusively on helping children feel comfortable and safe; the middle phase is designed to assess disclosures in indirect ways (or more direct ways, if children have spoken or revealed relevant issues in their play); and finally, the last three or four sessions are used to either say goodbye to children (termination of assessment) or to discuss with them (or their parents, depending on the children's age) the outcome of assessment and direction for treatment.

The goals of the assessment process include the following:

To determine the child's overall developmental functioning.
To identify current symptoms or problems.
To identify traumatic impact, if any.

To get an idea of the child's internal resources (coping strategies, ego strength).

To explore the child's perceptions of parental support and guidance.

To encourage appropriate parental support, nurturance, and guidance.

In order to achieve these goals, the assessment includes observation of several distinct categories of functioning and offers the child specific activities that have the potential of enhancing clinical data collection and development of a therapy relationship.

Observational Categories

We utilize the observational categories defined by Greenspan (1981) and differentiate children's functioning according to their developmental ages and stages. These domains include physical functioning, patterns of interactions (particularly attachment to important caretakers), thematic material, and fears and anxieties. We have added a few other observational categories for sexually abused children, including children's interest and understanding in sexuality (including the presence of sexual concerns and preoccupations or acting-out behaviors), as well as the presence of dissociative traits in their behavior or general expression.

Specific Assessment Strategies

Child-friendly atmospheres can immediately diffuse children's anxiety about coming to visit a therapist for the first time. When children attend therapy subsequent to investigative interviews, medical exams, or parent inquiries, clinicians are advised to minimize their reliance on verbal interviewing, and instead to provide an atmosphere of acceptance and permissiveness. Parents are encouraged to tell children that they will be meeting with therapists or counselors who work with children and who are interested in getting to know them a little, seeing how they're doing, and learning whether anything is causing them worries or concerns. When cases of child sexual abuse are already concluded legally, when children come to therapy after court procedures, or when children have made clear allegations of abuse, they can be told that their therapists or counselors work with lots of children who have been touched or hurt in their private parts. I sometimes encourage parents to tell their children that they can say as much or as little as they want, and that they will get to explore and decide on a number of play activities. The younger a child is, the fewer explanations are required. Parents are encouraged to bring their children to these assessment appointments the same way they would take them to a medical appointment or a school meeting.

Throughout our assessment process, we offer children opportunities to engage in some or all of the following activities (many of these are more fully described in Chapter Four):

Play genogram
Sand worlds or scenarios, and other forms of sand therapy
Color Your Feelings
Self-portrait
Kinetic Family Drawing
Symbol work
Verbal communication (often in combination with expressive techniques)
Puppet play, storytelling, and dramatic play
Completion of a paper-and-pencil instruments, such as the Trauma Symptom Checklist for Children (TSCC; Briere, 1996)

Depending on the age, gender, culture, and temperament of children, they may feel more comfortable with certain activities than with others. This comfort level will also be affected by the establishment of a therapy relationship (Landreth, 1991), personal perceptions of the relationship and activity known as therapy, competing interests outside therapy, and their parents' or caretakers' view of therapy as helpful in resolving the family crisis.

CASE EXAMPLE: GENE V.

Intake Session

Gene V. was a 7-year-old European American child referred to ACTS after he made a disclosure about child sexual abuse by a sports coach whom the family had known for years (and who had in fact coached Gene's older brother, Fred). During the intake session, the parents were distraught about Gene's alleged abuse, particularly about how their trust had been betrayed by this long-standing family friend. They felt confident that Gene would "be all right now that he had gotten things off his chest," but they were concerned about whether the abuse would result in later problems and whether their older child, Fred, had also been abused.

The parents described Gene as energetic, outgoing, and smart. Mrs. V. had a normal pregnancy with Gene, felt much more relaxed and prepared than she had with her first pregnancy, and described normal developmental milestones. She described the sibling relationship between Fred and Gene as "normal," with typical ups and downs. Mr. V. noted that there was some minor competition between the boys, but since Gene had decided to focus on soccer and Fred on baseball, they had gotten along much better.

Overall, this seemed like a functional, happy family. The parents seemed shocked that child sexual abuse had "hit our home," and they emphasized that they didn't want to "make too much" of the abuse but they also wanted Gene to "deal with everything" so that this wouldn't affect him in the future. Both parents denied any history of abuse themselves and noted a very lucky and uneventful life to date. The parents held hands throughout the intake session, became teary when discussing their son's sexual abuse, and gave each other a great deal of support and encouragement. Mr. V. had used the Internet to obtain information about child sexual abuse, and he seemed quite invested in the idea that early disclosure, parental support, and early but brief interventions would decrease the likelihood of long-term impact. I complimented both parents on their research and their willingness to bring Gene for an assessment to ensure that he had viewed the abuse realistically and didn't have any "hidden worries." When they asked about how much or little to say to Gene, or whether they should tell him about the coach's legal proceedings, I made the following statement in support of their balanced approach to date:

> "I'd like to follow your lead by encouraging you to continue to keep a balanced approach. Don't over- or underemphasize the abuse. Keep him informed of important things—for example, that the coach has confessed and will be going to court to see the judge—but, at the same time, I wouldn't talk about it constantly."

I went on to tell them that they should answer all his questions in a normal tone of voice, and that this would be an opportunity to role-model that the abuse was a permissible topic. It's always difficult to find the right balance in discussing abuse with children, but it's best to follow children's lead in this unless they either avoid all mention of the abuse or seem stuck in repetitive, indiscriminate discussions that seem obsessive in nature.

I then inquired about how much Fred had been told about the abuse. The parents reported that Fred knew about Gene's disclosures; in fact, Gene had told Fred about the allegations of abuse immediately after telling his parents. They also told me that when they had asked Fred about the coach, Fred did not seem surprised, but claimed he didn't know anything about the abuse at the time it was happening. We agreed that at some point it might be helpful to have a family meeting that included both boys. We scheduled an appointment for Gene, and I asked the parents simply to tell him that I work with lots of children who have made allegations of abuse, or have been abused, and that I am someone who talks with children and does "play therapy," which is a way of getting to know kids that includes playing with toys.

Session 1 with Gene

Gene was hesitant but receptive to meeting with me. He darted into my office when he spied the toys on one side of the room. He started playing with a toy helicopter that sat on a landing pad on top of a toy hospital. He was full of questions, and his eyes darted around the room. I stopped him and told him I'd give him a tour, since there was a lot to see. I talked about the two halves of my office: the half with the couch and chair "because some kids like to sit and chat," and the half with the toys "because I am a play therapist too, and there are lots of toys that we can play with." I took Gene around the room and showed him the sand trays, smooth sand, and miniatures, giving him directions for their use (see Chapter Four). When I showed him the miniature replica courtroom, he blurted out, "I might go to court to testify!" We then had the following exchange:

THERAPIST: Really?

GENE: Yep, Sargent Darrell told me I might have to go tell what Ed did to me!

THERAPIST: How do you feel about going to court to tell about Ed?

GENE: I don't know . . . OK, I guess . . . I didn't do anything wrong, he did!

THERAPIST: So you feel okay going to testify because you will be telling about something that Ed did wrong, not you.

GENE: Yep. Do you already know about Ed?

THERAPIST: Well, your mom and dad told me a little bit, but I thought I would get to know you and hear what you had to say.

GENE: Do I have to do that right now?

THERAPIST: Nope, unless you want.

GENE: I'll tell you later.

THERAPIST: Sure. Let me show you the rest of the room.

Gene reacted in a way that children can react when working with toys: He saw the miniature courtroom, and it immediately spurred him to talk about the fact that he might be going to testify in court. I don't know that he planned to talk about this, but I'm sure it must have been on his mind and didn't need too much stimulation to come forward. He was able to say about as much as he wanted; he asked me what I knew, and then chose to move on. I didn't press for more details and followed his lead.

Next, I showed Gene the hospital with helicopter and ambulance, the art and crafts supplies, the puppets, the dollhouse ("Yuck, that's for girls"), and some other miscellaneous things (e.g., a shield, cape, and Nerf sword; cars and trucks; expanding balls). He played mostly with the helicopter and set up elaborate rescue scenarios. I followed his directions and placed toys where he wanted, helped him, and generally participated as he instructed. He was sad to leave at the end of the session, and asked when he could return. We had made a good connection, and so far I had seen that his physical and emotional functioning was good, his verbal skills were excellent, and his imagination was vast and rich.

Session 2

When Gene came back to the second session, I told him he could play with anything he liked or talk to me about anything he chose. Gene wanted to play with the helicopter and hospital again, and this time he set up an elaborate story about a man who was drowning in the ocean (he used a sand tray to make an ocean scenario). The man had fallen off a boat and was yelling for help. The helicopter attendant got a call that someone was in trouble, and immediately gathered his rescue equipment and went to the scene of the drowning. Gene was very involved in this scene and played the roles of all the characters. He was particularly adept at having a dialogue between the two rescue attendants in the helicopter as they flew over the ocean and eventually spotted the "target" near his boat. The attendants then lowered a rescue stretcher and asked the man to grab hold. The man who was drowning couldn't seem to reach the stretcher, and finally the attendant yelled out, "Don't be afraid, sir. Just reach out and grab the stretcher. You'll be all right." The man was able to get into the stretcher after two tries, and the stretcher was pulled up. The man was then rushed to the hospital, placed in another stretcher, and carried to the emergency room. A male and a female doctor appeared quickly and asked a number of questions: "Are you all right?" "Can you speak?" "Can we call someone for you?" The man asked that his son be called to his side. His son appeared quickly thereafter, asking his dad why he had gone off fishing alone. Dad told him that he had not been able to awaken the boy, and the son replied, "Dad, you should have put cold water on me. I would have woken up and come with you." The dad apologized for leaving without him and then added, "Well, at least only one of us got in trouble, not both." The boy then thanked the helicopter attendants for rescuing his dad. Finally, he asked about the boat and whether they'd be able to go get it so that he and his dad might go fishing another time. The attendants acquiesced and got the boy and his dad their boat. "Next time," the boy said, "we won't go in dangerous waters!" The dad agreed.

Children's spontaneous stories are quite informative. As Engel (1995) states,

> We use stories to guide and shape the way we experience our daily lives, to communicate with other people and to develop relationships with them. We tell stories to become part of the social world, to know and reaffirm who we are. This is particularly true for young children. (p. 25)

Gene's story was quite revealing about his internal preoccupations. He created a scenario of imminent danger and rescue. He had an adult parent figure in danger of dying, but made sure that two rescue figures came and pulled him from the water in the nick of time. The father was then taken to the hospital for medical attention and, when asked who should be called, requested his son. His son assumed a parental role by chastising the father for going out alone without him (implying that if the son had been with him, he would not have been in danger). Finally, the boy made sure that their boat would be available for future adventures and assured the father that he, the boy, would make sure that they did not venture into dangerous waters (i.e., the boy would protect the father). In short, Gene's story seemed to demonstrate the importance of the father–son relationship, the journey they were on together; and their mutual dependence. Given the fact that Gene had just been abused by a trusted caretaker and was not rescued by his father, it was interesting to note that the boy's protection of the father might have been a projection of what Gene wished his father had done. The sequence of play ended with the boy promising to take care of the father and keep them both out of harm's way, perhaps revealing Gene's desire to be more self-sufficient in the future in order to keep himself (and his father) safe. Children often use storytelling as Gene did—that is, as a way of addressing some of their hidden concerns in a cushioned way. Storytelling opportunities are ample in play therapy and have been well discussed (Burns, 2005; Engel, 1995).

Session 3

At the time of the third session, Gene had just begun school and had lots to say about his new teachers, his friends, his new school clothes, and his new bike. He talked about the fact that he would be riding his bike to school, and that he had a new orange chain with a lock combination that only he knew. He seemed happy and a little distracted. He played just a little with the sand tray, the helicopter, and some clay, but was not focused or interested in prior activities. I told him that next time I would ask him to do a project with me, and he seemed agreeable.

Session 4

In the fourth session, I took a large sheet of easel paper and drew a large genogram (McGoldrick & Gerson, 1985; De Maria, Weeks, & Hof, 1999) of Gene's family (mother, father, and brother). We noted his grandparents as well; both grandmothers were living, and both grandfathers were dead. His Uncle James was staying with them for a while, so we included him in the genogram, as well as Gene's best friends or any other important people in his life. He asked cautiously what I meant by "important people in his life."

> THERAPIST: Well, anyone that has been important to you—anyone who has been in your life and that you've had a relationship with that you think of as important.
>
> GENE: (*Hesitating, and then speaking in a low voice*) Well, I knew Ed for a long time. He used to be my friend . . .
>
> THERAPIST: You can include Ed if you wish.
>
> GENE: I'm going to put him over here (*indicating a spot far removed from the family*).
>
> THERAPIST: How long did you know Ed?
>
> GENE: Since I was about 5 years old . . . he used to come to my house all the time, and he used to coach Fred.
>
> THERAPIST: Oh, so he was your coach and your brother's coach.
>
> GENE: Yeah, but he didn't do anything bad to Fred.
>
> THERAPIST: Ed didn't do anything bad to Fred? How do you know that?
>
> GENE: Because Fred told me so . . .
>
> THERAPIST: So you have asked your brother if Ed did anything bad to him?
>
> GENE: Yeah, he only did bad things to me.
>
> THERAPIST: (*Taking a chance*) What bad things did Ed do to you, Gene?
>
> GENE: You know . . .

THERAPIST: Well, I'm not really sure what you mean by "bad things."

GENE: My mom told me that you see kids who had bad things happen to them.

THERAPIST: I do. Lots of kids who come to see me have had people touch them in their private parts.

GENE: That's what Ed did to me. He touched me in my private parts.

THERAPIST: Yep, sometimes grownups do that. And you know what, Gene? (*Gene looks up*) Grownups who touch kids on their private parts have problems, and it is not okay for them to do that. Most grownups don't do that, just the ones that have problems.

GENE: (*Teary-eyed and speaking in a soft voice*) How come he did that?

THERAPIST: It's hard to know why . . . have you asked yourself that question?

GENE: I think it's because he's weird.

THERAPIST: Some grownups who touch kids' private parts do seem weird, I know, because they have problems in their heads that make them decide it's okay to touch kids in their private parts.

GENE: (*Looking up*) Yeah, he needs some help, and I hope he goes to jail.

THERAPIST: What kinds of feelings do you have about Ed?

GENE: I think he should go to jail!

THERAPIST: And when you say that, what feeling do you have?

GENE: I'm mad at him!

THERAPIST: So one of the feelings you have is that you're mad at him. What other feelings do you have?

GENE: Well, I feel sorry for him that he's so weird.

THERAPIST: So you have some angry feelings and some sorry feelings.

GENE: Yeah.

THERAPIST: It also looks like you and your family have known him for a long time, and you and your family probably liked him at one time.

GENE: Yeah, he used to come over for dinner, and he brought me and Fred some cool stuff. He used to be nice to us sometimes.

THERAPIST: That makes it confusing, doesn't it, because sometimes he was nice to you and your family, and other times he was touching your privates and that wasn't okay.

Finally Gene asked, "What is the project you wanted to do?" He had talked enough, and it was time to move on. "Thanks for reminding me," I said. The project was a play genogram (Gil, 2003c). I told him, "I'd like you to pick a miniature from all the choices on the shelves that best shows your thoughts and feelings about each person in your family, including yourself. Once you pick out each miniature, bring it over and place it on the square or circle where it belongs." Gene got up and started looking around: "It can be anything?" "Anything at all," I replied. His first choice was a figure for his brother, and he smiled and said under his breath, "This is a good one, this is a good one." Next, he selected a miniature for his mother, his father, and his Uncle James. He then chose a miniature for his two best friends, and finally asked if he had to pick something for Ed. I told him if he wanted to try to find a miniature for Ed, that would be fine. "That one might be hard," I added, "because it seems you have a lot of different thoughts and feelings about him." Gene looked hard and picked two figures for Ed. I then asked him for permission to take a picture, and not only did he agree, but he took the picture himself (see Figure 2.1). I also told him that maybe in the next session we would take a closer look at his miniatures, since we were almost out of time this session. "I have an idea," he said. "We can use the picture to put everything down just the way it is now." "Great idea," I said, comfortable with his interest in this task.

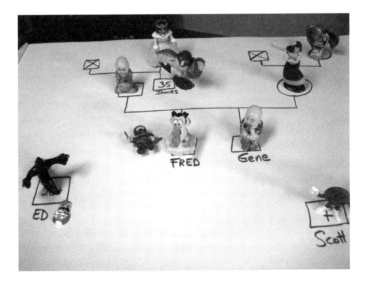

FIGURE 2.1. Individual play genogram.

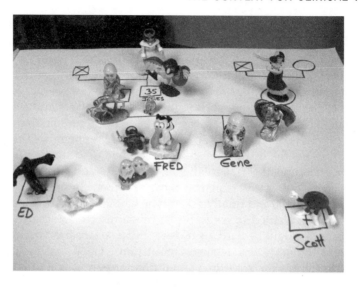

FIGURE 2.2. Fred's new miniature.

Session 5

Before the fifth session began, I put the large sheet of easel paper on the desk, and I printed Gene's picture out and placed it next to the sheet of paper. When Gene came in, he quickly began to find his miniatures and place them on the squares and circles. "I want a new one for my brother," he said, and placed a different miniature for Fred. "Wow," I said, "Fred sure gets some special miniatures." Gene asked, "Can I show him the picture?" "Sure, if you want. It's your picture, and you can show whoever you like."

I then told Gene that I had another part of the project to do today, and I asked him to find a miniature that best showed his thoughts and feelings about his relationship with each person on the genogram page. I clarified for him what that meant, and then he proceeded to place miniatures between himself and each person on the genogram (see Figure 2.2). He then talked briefly about his choices. I listened to Gene carefully as he was able to describe his intricate feelings by using symbols. Gene was also revealing more and more about himself in this partially defended way. Finally, before our session ended, I did a quick check of Gene's comfort level and then made a further request regarding the genogram:

> "Gene, you've done great picking miniatures and letting me know about your choices. Let me ask you one more thing. I'd like your dad

and mom [I pointed to the miniatures on the page] to say something to Ed about his touching your private parts. See what they might want to say to him about what he did."

Gene responded immediately to this request. Using the mother miniature first, he stated, "You are *not* welcome to my house any more, and I will *not* be cooking dinners for you! I hope you miss a whole bunch of my cooking!" Then Gene grabbed the Fred miniature, went up to the Ed miniature, and pushed it down. As Fred, he yelled, "Don't you mess with my little brother any more, hear me? I'll come and kick your butt!" Next, Gene grabbed the father miniature and went over and said:

> "I know you're a sick, sick man . . . it says so in the computer that you're sick, but you're never setting foot in my house again and I think you're evil for hurting Gene so much, especially because he liked you so much and looked up to you like you were an uncle, almost . . . I don't wish you bad things in jail, but I hope you can't eat that junk food you like so much and that you get very skinny and learn your lesson, and we better not see you hanging around other kids either!"

After Dad had said his piece, Gene sat back in his chair. He looked sad and said, "I wish he hadn't done those things to me." "I wish he hadn't either," I said. He cried a little, and I told him it was okay to cry and feel sad and have lots of feelings. "OK," he said, "I forgot to have my Uncle James say something." "Oops, that's right, a couple of people haven't said anything to Ed." Gene looked at me and realized that Uncle James wasn't the only one who hadn't spoken to Ed; he hadn't either! He took the Uncle James miniature and the Gene miniature, and he moved them together so that they faced the Ed miniature. "This is my real uncle," Gene said as himself, "and he's a good guy who is nice to me all the time, and he would never do weird things like you did. He's here to tell you something important." Then Gene spoke for the Uncle James miniature: "I just want you to know that you can't go around pretending to be a good guy and then mess up a kid's head. I want you to know that from now on, I'm the only uncle in this kid's life, and you won't be a part of our family any more." "*Yeah*," Gene said as himself, in a stronger voice. "You're not a real part of my family, only my dad and Uncle James!" He then stopped and said, "Okay, then, we told him!" "Yep," I said, "you and your Uncle James and everyone in your family have told Ed some of the feelings you have about his touching your privates." I then noted it was time to stop the session, and Gene asked for a new picture (which he took). The parents called after a few days to tell me that Gene had talked to the family about the play genogram. In fact, he had asked each family member to use his or her miniature to go talk to Ed, and he had told them what to say. Everyone in the family found this exercise very liberating, and the parents thanked me. I told them in reply that they had an exceptionally bright child who was confronting his fears directly and who was responding very well to a very difficult experience.

Session 6

When Gene came to session 6, I asked him if he would fill out a paper-and-pencil questionnaire, the TSCC. This instrument is particularly sensitive to symptoms commonly associated with traumatic experiences, such as anxiety, depression, dissociation, and sexual concerns. Gene asked me about some of the questions and what they meant, and I read them back to him and asked what he thought they might mean. He then used his pencil to endorse an answer for each question. The findings revealed only one area for attention: that of sexual concerns. Like many sexually abused boys, Gene seemed to have some confusions or worries about sexuality. In my experience, some young boys worry about homosexuality when they have been sexually abused by males; other worries may have to do with unwanted erections or sudden interest in masturbatory behaviors, particularly when these behaviors haven't been of particular interest in the past.

I talked to Gene directly about the results of the TSCC ("the questions you answered on the long sheet of paper"), and I printed out a grid that he could look at (this is often useful for children and adolescents to see). I showed him that the slight spike on the grid meant that he might be a little worried about sex. He looked shy when I said that, and then I asked if he knew what "sex" meant. He nodded affirmatively, although I made a mental note to ask his parents what they had taught Gene about sexuality so far in his young life. I asked Gene what he thought about when he thought of sex, and he said, "Touching private parts and being naked." I thought it best to elaborate once I talked to his parents. I then asked Gene if there was anyone that he felt he could talk to about sex. He replied, "Not really." I asked more specifically, "If you had a question about sex or about changes in your body or touching yourself (which, by the way, is normal) or anything like that, who would you ask?" He thought for a long time and said, "I guess my dad." I asked if he had ever had a talk with his dad about sex, and he said, "No." I told Gene that I would like to ask his dad to have a conversation with him if that was OK. Gene said that it was.

We then went on to play a board game (the Talking, Feeling, Doing Game; Gardner, 1973). When we got to the question "What's the worst thing a parent can do to a child?", Gene noted, "The worst thing anybody can do to a child is to touch him on his private parts." This gave me an opening to talk to Gene some more about how much this was on his mind and whether it popped into his mind often or a little. We used a rating scale of 0–10 to list the feelings he had about the abuse (anger, sadness, confusion, fear), and he rated how he felt when the abuse was going on and how he felt now. Regarding his feelings of anger and sadness, he indicated that his feelings were between 7 and 10 on the scale while the abuse was going on, and between 3 and 6 currently. He also noted that he currently felt confusion at a 5 and fear at a 3. As we continued the game, Gene got another question about anger, and this gave us another opportunity to talk about safe expression of anger. He seemed to be quite comfortable stating that he sometimes got angry (and that his parents also sometimes got angry). When I asked what his parents said or did to show their anger, he said that they talked in a "strict voice" and sent him to "time out." He reported that privileges (watching TV or playing outside) were suspended as punishment for wrongdoing, but he also stated that there was no hitting in the family.

Progress Report and Family Meeting about Sexuality

I made an appointment to talk with Gene's parents to give them a progress report. The most important issue was ensuring that the father would feel comfortable talking with his son about sexuality, and we discussed what Gene would need to know. I guided the parents through a discussion of positive messages about normative sexuality that they wanted to give to Gene; they made a decision to talk with Gene and Fred together, and even to invite Uncle James to participate in a male discussion of sexuality. The mother chose to allow her husband and sons to talk together, so that they wouldn't feel hesitant or embarrassed by her presence. Instead, she told her husband that she would come in at the end of the discussion, so that maybe she could hear the highlights of the conversation if the boys were comfortable with that.

The parents called me to report that the family meeting about sexuality had gone very well, with one notable exception: In the course of the discussion, Fred had broken down and admitted that he had heard that the coach had done something weird to another kid on the team. Fred felt terrible, because at the time he had dismissed the allegation and told his friends that they didn't know what they were talking about. Fred had harbored tremendous feelings of guilt since hearing about his brother's allegation; he had come to believe that if he had believed the rumors and had told someone about them, his brother wouldn't have been abused. Apparently the father and Uncle James had both been sensitive and responsive, and reassured Fred that there was no way he could have known what was going on. In fact, they wouldn't have believed the rumors at the time themselves, and the only one responsible for the abuse was Ed. Aside from that, apparently Gene was quite relieved to hear that when someone touches a penis, it does grow bigger; and that all boys and men touch themselves in private; and that it's perfectly normal for boys to be interested in how their bodies work. Gene had asked whether Ed was gay and whether that was why he had abused him, and the father stated that he didn't know. Gene then asked how people become gay, and the father said that people are more than likely born that way, but they don't catch it from someone else. Gene had then asked, "So I'm not gay?" Fred had piped up, "You are only gay if you like boys. You have a crush on Amanda, remember?" Gene denied that, but apparently it clarified his confusion. The father felt very positive about this meeting and told Gene and Fred they would talk about this more often, since there are so many issues that young boys need to know about. Both Mr. V. and James commented that they wished their parents had talked to them about sex when they were growing up, but some people just don't feel that comfortable discussing sex. Mrs. V. was also pleased that both her sons felt comfortable with recapping the meeting and giving her the highlights.

Session 7

In session 7, I asked Gene what was new, and he mentioned briefly that his father had talked to him and his brother about sex.

THERAPIST: How did that go?

GENE: Good . . Fred said that Ed had touched some other kid in our school.

THERAPIST: Oh. What did you think about that news?

GENE: I just thought he only did it to me . . .

THERAPIST: Well, when grown men have this problem, they tend to want to touch a lot of kids, not just one. He might have touched lots of other kids. I guess we won't know . . . How does it feel to you, knowing he might have touched other kids?

GENE: Well, not so good for them, but I'm glad that I'm not the only one.

THERAPIST: No, you're not alone. We see a lot of kids here who have been touched or hurt in their privates.

GENE: Do you see other boys?

THERAPIST: Yes, I do. As a matter of fact, sometimes when we have about four or five boys, we have a group for them so that they can talk together . . . I was thinking I might invite you to come to the group.

GENE: Oh, no . . . I don't want to talk to other kids.

THERAPIST: What do you think other kids would do or say?

GENE: They would laugh at me.

THERAPIST: Oh, so you worry that kids might laugh at you or make fun of you. Most kids are a little worried or shy about coming to group. Then when they come to group, they find that everybody has been through the same thing, and most of the time they don't laugh at each other . . . Maybe we'll talk some more about groups later.

GENE: Okay, but I don't *have* to come if I don't want to . . . ?

THERAPIST: That's right, you don't *have* to come if you don't want to, but we would probably ask you to try it out first so you could make a decision.

Gene then asked what we were going to do today, and I said that for part of the time I wanted to do an art project with him, and the rest of the time he could decide what to do.

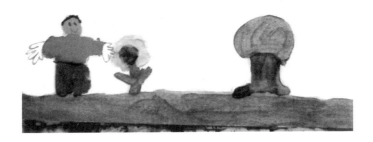

FIGURE 2.3. Gene's self-portrait.

I asked Gene to "draw a picture of yourself" (Malchiodi, 1998; Oster & Gould Crone, 2004). He said he wasn't a "good drawer," and I said that whatever he drew would be just fine with me. I gave him a pencil and a piece of paper, and he focused on the task quite easily. His drawing (see Figure 2.3) had no significant features. It was developmentally on target; it showed some interest in detail, good perception of body, a well-integrated picture, and a happy expression on his face. Gene also drew a cloud and the sun overhead. When I asked how he liked his picture, he said, "Pretty good. It came out good." He took it home to show his parents, but asked if I wanted to take a picture of it first. He again chose to take the picture himself. He then chose to spend the rest of our appointment time exploring the office, playing pick-up sticks, looking at the miniatures on the shelf, and rearranging some animals into categories. He noticed, for example, that someone had put a snake among the farm animals, and offered to put the snake on the shelf with the other snakes. This interest in order coincided with his mother's description of Gene as a "neat freak" who liked to keep his room fairly organized (in contrast to Fred, who let everything fall to the floor).

Session 8

In session 8, Gene and I first talked about the fact that this *was* session 8. I asked Gene if he remembered why he had first come to see me. He noted that his parents had brought him to see me because he had told about Ed. When I asked how he felt about telling, he said, "My parents told me I was brave to tell them, and I made the abuse stop." I commented that often telling someone about abuse is pretty hard to do. Gene stated in a firm voice, "Ed told me that if I told my dad, he might make me go live somewhere else." I wasn't sure exactly what Gene had said, so I clarified with him: "Ed or your dad would make you live somewhere else?" Gene seemed to approach this subject with trepidation. "Ed told me that my dad didn't really love me as much as Fred, and that he didn't want me to be born . . . Ed said he would take me to live far away with him." As I listened, I thought about Gene's constant play with adult male figures, and about the various times we had mentioned his dad and I had noticed some indescribable subtlety in his responses. Our conversation continued:

THERAPIST: So Ed tried to keep you from telling by putting some doubts in your head about your dad.

GENE: Yeah.

THERAPIST: Ed tried to make you think that your dad didn't love you that much.

GENE: Yeah.

THERAPIST: Hmmmm. That's a lot for you to have on your mind . . . that's a pretty big worry. (*Gene nods; pause*) What happened when you told your parents about Ed?

GENE: (*After some thought*) They told me I was brave and it was good that I told . . . My dad got mad at Ed.

THERAPIST: Your mom and dad were happy that you told them about what was going on, and then they got mad at Ed and called the police.

GENE: That's right.

THERAPIST: Sounds like Ed was wrong.

GENE: Yeah. Maybe he was trying to trick me so I wouldn't tell.

THERAPIST: That's probably the way it was. Grownups who tell kids to keep secrets from their parents are usually trying to trick them or get away with something they know isn't right. (*Gene is playing close attention*) Let me ask you a question, Gene. (*Gene looks up, making direct eye contact*) Did Ed ever touch your private parts in front of your parents or your brother or other kids?

GENE: No. He always took me somewhere and locked the door.

THERAPIST: Why do you think he did that, Gene?

GENE: I don't know. I didn't like it when other people left.

THERAPIST: You didn't like being alone with him, but he only touched your private parts when you two were alone.

GENE: Yeah.

THERAPIST: Do you have any guesses about why he wanted to be alone with you?

GENE: Yeah, because he wanted to touch my privates!

THERAPIST: That's right, but he already knew he was doing something wrong, because he only did it when there was no one else around to see what he was doing or to stop him.

GENE: (*Thinks about this for a while; pushes holes into a piece of clay he is holding*) He was doing something bad, and he knew it was bad. (*Therapist nods*) He told me that my parents knew what he was doing, and that all kids like it.

THERAPIST: Yep, people who touch kids make up lots of different excuses for what they do . . . it can be confusing for kids.

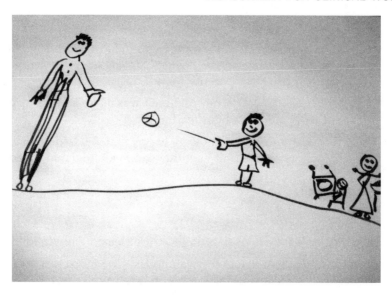

FIGURE 2.4. Kinetic family drawing.

Gene had had enough at this point and asked if he could play. I told him that he could, but I wanted to take a few more minutes for another art project. He agreed readily and went to get the pencil from the desk. "Today I'd like you to draw a picture of you and your family doing something together—some kind of action." He drew quickly this time (perhaps so he could move on to playing more freely), and he again noted that it was a "good picture." He drew a picture of himself and his dad playing catch while his mom cooked hot dogs and Fred watched television (see Figure 2.4). "I like playing catch with my dad," he said affirmatively, and asked to play a game called Mankala that we had played one other time.

At the end of the session, I thanked Gene for talking with me about all the things that Ed had told him and how he felt confused. I told him that I was going to think some more about how to help him with these feelings, and we would probably meet with everybody in his family at some point. I told him that we would also have a couple more individual meetings, and he asked, "How come?" I reminded him that I had told him and his parents at the start that I would meet with him for about 10–12 times, and then I would tell him what I thought might be helpful for him. He said, "Oh, yeah." I had already decided that it would be beneficial for him to attend group therapy.

Session 9

The next session, Gene came in announcing that it was session 9. He asked if we could have another five times together. I told him that my job was to get to know him a little bit and try to figure out what I thought would help him the most. I asked him if his parents had ever taken him to the doctor when he had a fever or a sore throat. He told me that he had had an operation once (ear tubes) and that it had hardly hurt at all. I told him that doctors try to figure out how to help kids when they are sick. I then told him that I was also a doctor, and my job was to help kids who had been touched in their private parts and figure out what would help kids the most. Gene was quiet as he began playing with clay, making a big pig (he had just gone to a county fair the day before). I reminded Gene that I had told him we would meet for about 10–12 times for me to figure out what I thought would be helpful to him (although sometimes fewer sessions are needed). I also reminded him that I would probably make some recommendations to his parents about future therapy. Gene remembered, and asked if I had already talked to his parents; once he understood that I had not, he listened attentively to what I had to say. I continued, "I have two suggestions for you and your family. The first is that we meet together with your family so that we can talk about what happened, because this is something that happened to you *and* to them. Everyone

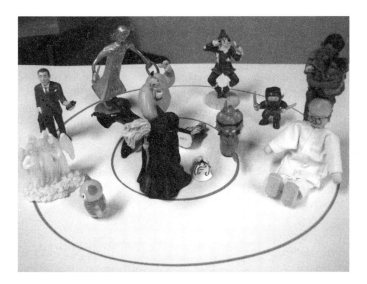

FIGURE 2.5. Circles project.

has feelings about it." Gene interrupted, "Will Fred come too?" "Yep, everyone in your family." "What else?" he asked. "The second suggestion I have is that you come to a group for boys who have been sexually abused." Gene made a face and asked how many boys would be in the group and what day of the week and time it would be (he was worried about a possible conflict with his baseball practice). I then asked him to decide what he wanted to do in our last individual meeting, and he went from one toy to another, as if saying goodbye to his favorite things. He asked to make a drawing at the end of our time and quickly drew a big sun with a smile and sunglasses. He added a bubble to the top of the picture that said "Goodbye." I scheduled a meeting with Gene's family for the following week. Gene expressed no particular feelings about coming to see me with his family.

Family Session

In our first family session, I asked everyone in the room to go and find a miniature that best showed his or her thoughts and feelings about the sexual abuse by Ed. I brought a round table to the center of the room, and the family was led by an enthusiastic Gene to the part of the room with the miniatures. He excitedly told his brother about the miniatures, and his parents looked around with curiosity. Gene's mother asked for clarification—in particular, whether she had to limit herself to one miniature. I told her she could do whatever she wanted. As the parents and the boys grabbed the miniatures, I asked them to place them on the small circle in the center. It took them about 15 minutes to complete this project (see Figure 2.5). The miniatures were very expressive. Before the family members got comfortable in their chairs, I told them that there was a second part of this project. I told them now to pick a miniature that showed how they had dealt with the problem, what had helped them, and where they were at right now. I told them to hold on to these miniatures when they returned to their seats.

I began by thanking everyone for coming to see me. I had not met Fred before, and I gave him a special greeting, telling him I had heard lots of nice things about him from his parents and his brother. The boys smiled at each other.

I then talked to the family directly about Ed:

"I know that you've all been through a difficult time. You trusted this man Ed, and it turns out that he was hurting you behind your back and touching Gene in his private parts. As a grownup, I'm sure he knew that was wrong to do . . . When sex abuse happens in families, it affects everyone, and I want to make sure that everyone feels comfortable talking about it openly, since part of how this happened was that Ed tricked Gene and scared him into keeping quiet. [I noticed Gene look around at everyone when I said that.] I'm wondering if everyone knows about how tricky Ed was."

Mr. V. spoke about this right away: "Ed tricked Gene *and* he tricked Mom and me. We thought he was so nice and helpful, we took him into our family." I asked Gene how he felt, knowing that Ed had tricked his mom and dad and Fred. Gene replied, "He told me that you wouldn't want me any more." Mr. V. didn't quite understand what Gene said. "What do you mean?" he asked Gene. Gene looked at me and said, "You tell him." "You want me to tell him about how Gene tricked you?" "Yeah," he said. I turned to his family and said, "Apparently Ed told Gene that you, Mr. V., loved your other son more and you hadn't wanted Gene to be born." Mr. V. raised his voice: "What? What a jerk!" I asked Mr. V. to tell Gene what he thought about what Ed had said. Mr. V. grabbed Gene and hugged him:

"Your mother and I tried and tried to get another little boy in our family. We hoped you would be a little boy. We couldn't stop smiling for a week. Fred was excited too, because he didn't want a sister in his family. [Gene sank into his father's arms.] Ed was a big trickster . . . he was just trying to get away with doing something that is not OK. [Almost on cue, Mr. V. repeated something we had discussed:] Your private parts belong just to you, Gene, and no one can touch you there unless it's a doctor trying to keep you healthy or, when you were little, your mom and dad changing your diapers."

Gene smiled. Fred added, "Yeah, he got toilet-trained a little while ago." The family laughed. Mrs. V. then said, "Honey, you did the right thing telling us about Ed. He was just trying to keep you from telling because he knew he would get in trouble. Probably everything he told you was a lie." Mr. V. added, "He's going to be punished so he learns his lesson." I echoed Mr. V.: "What Ed did is not OK, and it's important that he learn his lesson so he never hurts another kid." Fred asked whether Ed would get in trouble for the other kid that he touched, and I said I didn't know. Mr. V. then took a deep breath and said, "Your mom and I are crazy about you and your brother. We love you a lot." The father seemed much more warm and expressive than any other time I had seen him—almost as if he had risen to the occasion.

I then noted that it was important for everyone in the family to be able to talk or show each other whatever feelings they had about Ed, because they had all initially cared for him and later been tricked by him. This might have generated a range of feelings and thoughts, such as betrayal, compassion, anger, shame, guilt, and so forth. At that point I told them we'd return to the project, and I asked them to say a little about the miniatures they had placed on the table. The family members participated fully, talking about the choices they had made. It was a lively discussion.

Then I asked the boys and their parents to take turns and put the second miniature each person had had chosen on the outer circle. Fred began, and Gene was the last one to take a turn. Slowly but surely, they focused on how things were better now, what they had learned about how strong their family was, and how they viewed Ed (they felt sorry for him that he had a problem, but they wanted him punished for the hurt he had caused).

Recommendations, Further Treatment, and Comments

At the end of this session, I made my recommendations. I noted that although Gene was doing very well, I thought he could benefit from talking with other boys his age who had also been touched in their private parts (sexually abused). I also thought that we could meet again for a few more family therapy sessions, since they did so well talking with each other. Both parents seemed relieved to hear that Gene was doing well, and they agreed to bring Gene to a few group therapy sessions so that Gene could decide whether he liked it or not. I emphasized that it was important for Gene to make a choice about this after he came a few times and saw for himself what it would be like. Gene followed through by coming to the first two sessions reluctantly. After that, he seemed very happy to participate with the other boys in the group and blossomed into an effective leader. I met with the parents a few more times and talked with them on the phone over the next few months to clarify or discuss Gene's behaviors, successes, and struggles.[2]

Gene and his family illustrate a typical extended developmental assessment (and treatment) process with a resilient child and a strongly

---

[2] Parents often struggle with viewing new problems or concerns within the framework of earlier abuse. For example, when children get poor grades, develop a behavioral problem like stealing or lying, or experience a nightmare, parents tend to wonder whether these are consequences of the abuse. Distinguishing between normal developmental challenges and the aftereffects of abuse can be perplexing and will probably require careful attention to the type and persistence of the problem.

supportive family. His abuse had been very stressful, but Gene had told someone before the abuse turned more chronic or more severe. Not all assessments have this level of family participation, and not all children engage in dialogues as readily as Gene did. However, an extended developmental assessment is an attempt to understand the child's experience, to determine how he or she is managing the crisis, and to allow the clinician to make an informed treatment plan. Gene was a healthy child who utilized both verbal and nonverbal strategies to externalize his emotional responses, confusion, and concerns regarding the abuse and his family's responses. Gene's family also had many strengths that advanced Gene's understanding and processing of his experience. In many ways, this example demonstrates how well a crisis can be resolved when a family works together to face and resolve difficult life events.

SUMMARY

Abused children, especially sexually abused children, do not usually seek out treatment on their own; they may be referred either after disclosures of abuse have been made, or after emotional or behavioral problems have been identified by professionals or parents. Abused children may experience many obstacles to talking about their abuse, including linguistic or developmental limitations, fear of punishment, threats by abusers, or difficulties brought about by emotions such as shame or guilt. In addition, abused children may undergo multiple investigatory interviews with different professionals, and by the time of their first therapy appointment may be resistant to talking yet again about their abuse. For all these reasons, and because children usually find it easier to communicate by nonverbal or indirect verbal means, it is useful to invite children to participate in play-based, initially nondirective assessments designed to allow them the time to develop security and familiarity with the assessment/treatment process and with their clinicians. Their art, storytelling, use of metaphorical language, and use of miniatures or other toys will reveal a great deal about their current functioning, concerns, preoccupations, and questions. A trained clinician documents and chronicles a child's movement through the assessment phase, taking special note of the child's play themes, repetitions, and selection or avoidance of activities. During the assessment, the clinician also begins to observe the child's general functioning, patterns of relationships, anxieties, fears, and presence of symptomatic behavior. More importantly, the clinician gathers information (through both structured and unstructured methods) that allows for an

understanding of the child's phenomenological experience—that is, the inimitable meaning the child is making of what has happened.

As I have described at the beginning of this chapter, the assessment and treatment of abused (especially sexually abused) children and their families require a departure from traditional psychotherapy. Because children's disclosures set a complicated legal and clinical process into motion, mental health professionals must integrate nontraditional services within a multidisciplinary framework that maintains a focus on safety and advocacy. Probably the features that distinguish work with child maltreatment in general and sexual abuse in particular from work with generic mental health problems include the focus on risk factors and safety, as well as the need to work within a larger system of helping professionals. Specifically, clinicians in these cases may find themselves navigating case management issues that may feel unfamiliar and stressful. Families that experience child sexual abuse, particularly intrafamilial incest, may have a host of stressors and concrete problems; clinicians may need to function in an advocacy role to access and arrange for a host of collateral services (home-based services, hotlines, respite care, parenting classes, etc.). Initial clinical efforts usually focus on providing crisis intervention, assuring children's safety, decreasing risk factors, and assessing each child and family's unique therapy needs. Subsequent efforts tend to include coordination of community services, as well as referrals to particular therapy services (e.g., couple or family therapy and group therapy).

The extended developmental assessment is thus a structured approach that allows clinicians to evaluate children's overall functioning, identify symptomatic behaviors, assess the impact of trauma (if any), and assess children's phenomenological experience of the abuse (including their perceptions of parental support and guidance). At the same time, when children are able to converse and express their needs clearly, clinicians will take steps to address immediate or urgent matters—particularly issues such as suicidality. The extended developmental assessment utilizes a combination of directive and nondirective strategies in order to maximize engagement with children of diverse personalities and temperament, gender, culture, and developmental status. The initial phase of such assessment is nondirective, with a shift to a more directive stance during the middle phase. A clinician makes substantial efforts to create a safe and comfortable environment for a child and to establish a predictable therapeutic relationship. These two variables will maximize the child's potential to utilize the full benefits of treatment.

An extended developmental assessment lasts between 10 and 12 sessions, at the end of which a clinician should be able to determine therapy plans with specific, measurable goals and clear time frames. In some

cases (such as the one described in this chapter), where the traumatic impact is relatively low and where both the child and family have the internal and external resources to obtain maximum benefit from the assessment process, little or no further treatment (other than booster or follow-up sessions) may be required.

3

Guidelines for Integrated Treatment

Jerome Kagan [cited in Efran, Mitchell, & Gordon, 1998] described development as being similar to the growth of a tree. Step by step, stage by stage, the child builds upon what came before. From a family and community perspective, the roots of the tree can be dense, thick, and supportive or weak, fragmented, and fragile. The strength of a child's roots and stem symbolize the attachment the child experienced in his early years. A strong, fixed stem and widespread, deep roots can withstand heavy winds and temporary droughts. The roots and the stem form the basis for the branching and foliage, thick or thin. The foliage, in turn, provides the nutrients to rebuild and maintain the tree.

—R. KAGAN (2004, p.9)

Reisman (1971, cited in Reisman & Ribordy 1993, p. 7) defined "psychotherapy" as "the communication of person-related understanding, respect, and a wish to be of help." The importance of the relationship, and of positive contact within the relationship, is paramount. Reisman and Ribordy (1993) further note:

Person-related understanding refers to all communications that attempt to comprehend the client's or other person's thoughts, feelings and behaviors, regardless of whether this understanding is based on Freudian, Skinnerian, or any other theory. *Respect* denotes a positive regard for the individual's dignity, rights, uniqueness, and capacities for constructive change. *A wish to be of help* is simply that, and it implies that the professional is motivated by the desire to assist the person; this is usually assumed to be the case in the therapist–client relationship. (p. 8; emphasis in original)

Given the extensive evidence that child abuse and neglect contribute to a range of physical, behavioral, emotional, and psychological problems in children's development, and that chronic abuse can create trauma-related concerns and developmental delays, it is generally considered appropriate and necessary for abused children to receive a course of psychotherapeutic treatment.

The field of child psychotherapy is fairly new. It was only as recently as the mid-1980s that a consensus was reached about the effectiveness of psychotherapy for children; the conclusion was that it "reduced the severity of symptoms, speeded the process of healing or recovery, and helped people acquire new techniques for coping with personal problems" (Reisman & Ribordy, 1993, p. 11). However, Reisman and Ribordy add that "there is still much . . . that needs to be learned from research about enhancing the effectiveness of these procedures, including about when psychotherapy should be offered" (p. 11).

The 1990s and the early 2000s have witnessed an increased interest in evidence-based therapies. In the introduction to their vital book *Treatments That Work with Children*, Christophersen and Mortweet (2001) state that "The dearth of intervention studies in clinical child psychology only adds to the burden of clinicians who are responsible for the treatment of children" (p. 4). Prior (1996) notes that "there is no agreed-upon model of conceptual understanding and therapeutic practice that most clinicians would adhere to, and that would form a framework for shared assumptions, practices, and interpretive ideas" (p. 5). This prompts Prior to speculate that clinicians "are struggling to find their way, with little to guide them and certainly no comprehensive model with which to work" (p. 5). In the present chapter, when a specific type of therapy is currently considered "evidence-based," I have described it as such; to date, however, few approaches to therapy have been thoroughly enough studied with abused and traumatized children to justify this description.

There is far less uncertainty about the psychological effects of child abuse (especially sexual abuse) and the general emotional and behavioral problems that result (Berliner & Elliott, 2002). Kendall-Tackett, Williams, and Finkelhor (1993) conducted a meta-analysis of existing methodologically sound research studies on effects of child sexual abuse to discern whether a "profile" exists. They found no such profile but, did assert that four cluster areas appeared with vigor across studies: symptoms of PTSD; depression; general aggression; and sexual concerns, sexual preoccupations, or sexual aggression. These cluster areas include a variety of symptoms that may be more or less visible in different children. For example, in our client population at ACTS, we note presenting problems such as fear and anxiety; nightmares; generally heightened emotionality; temper tantrums and oppositional or provocative behaviors; sadness; suicidal ideation; aggression toward peers or property; boundary violations; sexual acting out; attachment problems; and a range of self-esteem and self-image concerns. It's particularly important to note the growing concern over attachment disturbances, especially reactive attachment disorder (Hanson & Spratt, 2000). We have also noted that younger children referred to our program have a more limited range of acting-out behaviors, whereas their adolescent counterparts may run away, use alcohol or drugs, engage in risky sexual behaviors, and engage in self-injurious behaviors (e.g., cutting). The list of symptoms that can be experienced by abused children is lengthy and disturbing, but definitely well documented (Berliner & Elliott, 2002).

Since the early 1990s, many authors have described treatment methodologies for abused children (more often than not, sexually abused children). These authors appear to concur on areas that require treatment (see, e.g., Kagan, 2004; Osofsky, 2004b; Stien & Kendall, 2004; Steele & Raider, 2001; Brohl, 1996; Ciottone & Madonna, 1996; Deblinger & Heflin, 1996; Karp & Butler, 1996; Prior, 1996; Friedrich, 1990, 2002a; Cattanach, 1992; Gil, 1991). However, some of these authors specify a particular treatment strategy—for example, Deblinger and Heflin's (1996) use of cognitive-behavioral therapy (CBT) or Steele and Raider's (2001) sensory integration model—whereas other authors seem to utilize a broad base of theories and approaches in order to best address the wide range of presenting problems in abused children. My own belief is that the authors of clinical articles, chapters, or books may find it more relevant and useful to specify problems that need to be addressed in treatment than to presume to instruct professional audiences in one particular theory or approach for resolving particular problems. Specifying a treatment problem and allowing clinicians to utilize their own theoretical frameworks and congruent strategies may be more effective than suggesting theories and strategies that some clinicians may resist. However, to give readers an impression of the literature in this area, I briefly describe the treatment goals and approaches advocated by many of the authors cited above. (Deblinger and Heflin's [1996] CBT model is discussed in Chapter Five, and a description of my own treatment approach follows the literature review.)

TREATMENT GOALS AND APPROACHES:
A BRIEF REVIEW OF THE LITERATURE

Friedrich (1990) cited Finkelhor and Browne's (1985) traumagenic factors—traumatic sexualization, stigmatization, betrayal, and powerlessness—as pivotal to the understanding of sexually abused children's treatment needs. He also specified the following important goals: (1) making meaning of the abuse experience; (2) helping children to view themselves more accurately; (3) decreasing the likelihood of further abuse; (4) providing the children with an experience that they view as both positive and meaningful in the future if the need arises; and (5) addressing specific behavioral goals. In subsequent work, Friedrich (2002a) has prioritized four treatment goals to be addressed—attachment, emotional dysregulation, self-perception, and family relationship—and designed specific goals and treatment modalities for each category. These goals are supported by current scientific research, which notes problems regulating emotion and arousal (hyperactivity, impulsivity, and attention problems), chaotic patterns of relating to others, and damage to self-concept and identity (alteration in system of beliefs) (Stien & Kendall, 2004).

Brohl (1996) divides treatment into the three stages of confusion, reorganization, and integration. In the first stage, the therapist forms an emotional attachment, reassures children, and reinforces positive changes. In the second, the therapist focuses on body safety and feelings of unsafety, guides children through unsafe moments, and again reinforces positive changes. In the third, the therapist discusses trauma, teaches new coping skills, and facilitates children's resolution of trauma, once again reinforcing positive changes.

Karp and Butler (1996) work within a treatment model with four phases that include attention to specific issues. Phase 1 addresses image building, goal setting, therapeutic trust, expressing feelings, and discussing boundaries; phase 2 explores the trauma by addressing trust and safety, secrets, memories, nightmares, and "monsters"; phase 3 works on self-reparation, including letting go of guilt/shame and working through "stuck" feelings; and phase 4 works on developing an orientation to the future and reviewing what's been learned.

Kagan's (2004) work focuses on building healthy attachments and utilizing narrative approaches to identify and foster real-life heroes, so that traumatized children can build the interpersonal resources needed to integrate painful memories without repetition of trauma behaviors. He provides a life story workbook, which is used to promote a range of creative arts, psychodrama, and other guided interactions that help children "reexperience the components of early trauma within the embrace of a safe, nurturing relationship with a caring, committed adult" (p. 299). Kagan's focus on attachment stems from his belief that attachment is critical to children's development:

> Attachment forms the foundations for a child's future relationships, learning, and expectations. The strength of a child's attachment shapes his or her emotional regulatory system and fosters exploration and mastery, feelings of self-confidence, empathy, language development, reasoning processing, and the ability to manage and resolve conflict. (p. 9)

Ciottone and Madonna (1996) provide a detailed case study using the play therapy techniques advanced by Ginott (1959), which include constructs drawn from psychodynamics, learning theory, and cognitive development. In particular, Ginott emphasized the use of good boundaries and limit-setting as central to the therapeutic process (Ginott, 1961).

Although Ciottone and Madonna don't speak about specific *goals* in therapy, they do discuss basic *premises* that guide the therapy. Based on those premises, they note that the therapist's task "becomes one of helping a child achieve developmental advance in self-world relationships (i.e., increasingly differentiated and hierarchically integrated cognitive, affective, and valuative constructions of the physical, interpersonal, and sociocultural aspects of the environment) and develop correspondingly more advanced instrumentalities for transacting with the world thus structured" (p. 39). They encourage therapists to make available toys that facilitate communication in the area of concern; develop good rapport and trust, which in turn allows for areas of conflict and concern to emerge; maintain child–adult distinctions; remain mindful of the power dimension when reflecting upon the inferred meaning of play; understand that even helping gestures can be construed differently by children; provide good limits and boundaries; and monitor the degree of intimacy that is required.

Prior (1996) finds that working with the transference issues in the therapy relationship holds some promise. Through such work, children can learn to negotiate their own sense of blame and powerlessness, their need to reenact the abuse dynamics in order to protect themselves, and the basic disorganization of their psyches.

Cattanach (1992) tailors her therapy interventions to meet four basic needs for growth in children: the need for love and security; the need for new experiences; the need for praise and recognition; and the need for responsibility. Her play therapy model is designed to help abused children "make sense of [their] experience of abuse and find ways of functioning which do not re-process the patterns of the abusive relationship" (p. 41). To accomplish this, she utilizes four concepts: the centrality of play as children's way of understanding their world; children's achievement of individuation and separation through play; play as a symbolic process through which children can experiment, at a distance from the consequences of their choices in real life; and, finally, play as a therapeutic space in which the child defines who is "me" and "not me," and the place where creative life starts.

Steele and Raider (2001) described their sensory integration model in their book, *Structured Sensory Intervention for Traumatized Children, Adolescents, and Parents*. Their primary intervention strategies are reliving the incident (exposure), telling the story (trauma narrative), and reordering the experience in a manageable way (cognitive reframing). This approach is most congruent with trauma-focused play therapy (see Chapter Seven of the present book), in which children are encouraged to utilize play in order to externalize their areas of distress (exposure); to learn to tolerate and release affect (abreaction); and to compensate for injuries and create feelings of mastery (management and restoration of power).

In Osofsky's (2004b) edited text, she and her colleagues suggest developing and fostering therapeutic alliances with both the child and his or her parents, as well as "helping the child with transitions and changes in daily routines, encouraging the expression of strong and difficult emotions through play therapy, providing a safe and stable environment, and assisting the child to adopt more adaptive relationship models and interaction strategies" (Klapper, Plummer, & Harmon, 2004, p. 151). Osofsky and her colleagues promote a careful assessment of the parent–child relationship and utilize the parent–infant interaction procedure (developed by Crowell & Feldman, 1989) and the Parent Perception Interview (based on the Working Model of the Child Interview, developed by Zeanah & Benoit, 1995). They propose seven treatment goals: (1) promoting a return to normal development, adaptive coping, and engagement with present activities and future goals; (2) fostering a realistic response to threat; (3) maintaining regular levels of affective arousal; (4) building reciprocity of intimate relationships; (5) normalizing the traumatic response; (6) encouraging a differentiation between reliving and remembering; and (7) placing the traumatic experience in perspective (Weberman & Van Horn, 2004, pp. 124–125). In spite of the fact that the Osofsky (2004b) text is primarily about young traumatized children, these treatment principles can apply to older children and adolescents as well.

Finally, several authors have accentuated the need to pay attention to children's neurobiology (Stern, 2002; Stien & Kendall, 2004). Stien and Kendall focus specifically on traumatized children with complex PTSD. Basing their work on Herman's (1992) three-stage model of working with adult survivors, they set forth three analogous stages for treating children: (1) safety and stabilization (creating a safe, predictable environment, stopping self-destructive behaviors, and providing psychoeducation on trauma and its effects); (2) symptom reduction and memory work (reducing arousal and regulating emotion, finding comfort from others, tolerating affect, integrating emotions and accepting ambivalence, overcoming avoidance, improving attention and decreasing dissociation, doing memory work; and (3) work on developmental skills (enhancing problem-solving capacities, nurturing self-awareness, social skills training, and developing a value system). Stien and Kendall also discuss the importance of reconnecting to the body and attending to attachment problems.

A number of these authors encourage the use of play, metaphor, and art to promote therapy goals. Stien and Kendall (2004) describe the neurological basis for providing such interventions for traumatized children:

> ... because traumatic memories are often firmly lodged in the right hemisphere, children tend to be controlled by negative emotions ... and self-defeating behaviors. Thus an important goal of treatment is to help children process experience through as many modalities as possible (e.g., images, thoughts, emotions, sensations, and movement), and to design experiences that can activate both hemispheres, especially the left (e.g., experiences that stimulate positive emotions and encourage initiative and action). (p. 137)

Art, play, and sand therapies (discussed in Chapter Four of the present book) are all highly desirable as ways to stimulate both hemispheres of the brain but achieve this by first eliciting right hemisphere activity.

In his recent article on developmental trauma disorder (see Chapter One), van der Kolk (2005) further emphasizes the need for interventions that involve movement and pleasure:

> Complexly traumatized children need to be helped to engage their attention in pursuits that do not remind them of trauma-related triggers and that give them a sense of pleasure and mastery. Safety, predictability and "fun" are essential for the establishment of the capacity to observe what is going on, put it into a larger context, and initiate physiological and motoric self-regulation. [Moreover,] only after children develop the capacity to focus on pleasurable activities without becoming disorganized do they have a chance to develop the capacity to play with other children, engage in simple group activities, and deal with more complex issues. (p. 407)

For clinicians pursuing a neurobiological approach, Stien and Kendall (2004, pp. 135–136) recommend the following treatment goals:

- Restore the natural hierarchy in the brain by decreasing the reactivity of the stress response and enhancing the inhibitory capacities of the cortex.
- Create a physiological state that promotes healthy brain development through the modulation of emotion.
- Enhance integrative functions by helping children to process experience through various modes.
- Build, reorganize, and strengthen new brain circuitry through experiences that generate new ways of thinking, feeling, and behaving.

More purely psychological goals, adapted by Stien and Kendall from the International Society for the Study of Dissociation (ISSD) Task Force on Children and Adolescents (2000), include the following:

- Help children learn how to regulate their emotions.
- Promote acceptance of painful emotions.
- Promote the direct expression of feelings in healthy attachments and relationships.
- Help children to reduce symptomatic behavior (e.g., withdrawing or acting out).
- Desensitize traumatic memories and correct the faulty beliefs about life caused by traumatic events.
- Promote a unified identity by helping children achieve a sense of cohesiveness about their own thoughts, feelings, and behavior.
- Enhance motivation for growth and future success.

Goals for the family are also identified by Stien and Kendall (p. 136).

As noted in Chapter One, the most promising aspect of the current research on brain development is the focus on reparative potential of the brain. Ratey (2001) notes that new experiences are the most effective way to change the pattern of connections among nerve cells, networks, and systems. Stien and Kendall (2004) encourage clinicians to design a three-pronged approach and state:

> Although cognitive/behavioral interventions address problematic behaviors and help the child build new skills, psychodynamic interventions are needed to help integrate traumatic memories and emotions along with buried parts of the self. At the same time, the therapist must pay close attention to family interactions—sequences of action and reaction—to root out any that maintain and reinforce symptoms. (p. 139)

Length of treatment is yet another question on which clinical opinions vary. Some therapists recommend long-term treatment for children with complex trauma, while others encourage a time-limited, more brief approach. The ISSD Task Force on Children and Adolescents states that "it is appropriate to maintain an open-minded and hopeful stance about the possibility of rapid treatment even for the most severe presentation which has occurred in many cases" (p. 118).

It becomes apparent from reading this brief summary of treatment goals and approaches that most clinicians with experience in treating abused children arrive at similar conclusions about areas for attention. Although different theories and approaches are endorsed by different experts, it appears that an integration of approaches might serve children best as we struggle to engage them in trusting relationships, offer them psychoeducational information, address their problems in relating to others, and help them discuss or process their traumatic memories and phenomenological experiences.

My particular approach to integrated treatment has been developed through direct experience with children over the last three decades. I describe it in the remainder of this chapter.

INTEGRATED TREATMENT: GENERAL PRINCIPLES

Given the general consensus on broad areas for therapeutic attention, the following principles may assist toward the goals of restoring normative functioning; allowing children to express themselves in general and about their abuse in particular; restoring feelings of security and mastery; and helping children develop and utilize adaptive coping strategies and external resources in the future. Clinicians who work with abused children seem to agree that polarized responses—ones that either ignore/ avoid or overfocus on traumatic stressors—will not help toward necessary resolution and future orientation. A balanced approach will usually include careful assessments; short-term individual, group, or family treatments; and the continuing delivery of services as children grow and develop and as deemed necessary (Gil, 1991).

I rely on these general treatment principles as guideposts in my treatment of abused and traumatized children:

- Provide a child-friendly therapeutic setting in which children and their families receive timely and informed responses.
- Conduct a comprehensive assessment of each child and family, withholding assumptions and biases that might affect clinical goal setting and expectations for treatment outcome.

- Construct a genuine, respectful, trust-filled, earnest *relationship* with each child client and his or her family.
- Provide services within a coordinated multidisciplinary context that centers on the best interests of the child, while also maintaining an awareness of legal procedures, time frames, and outcomes.
- Ensure that all clinical interactions are sensitive to culture (Cohen, Deblinger, Mannarino, & de Arellano, 2001), gender (Friedrich, 1995), and developmental age and stage (Greenspan, 1997; Hewitt, 1999).
- Maintain a focus on contextual and systemic issues.
- Assist parents or other caretakers to understand and better manage their crisis situation and respond appropriately to their children.
- Provide therapeutic approaches and services that best match the learning styles of parents/caretakers and children.
- Make a balanced and realistic assessment of family strengths and vulnerabilities.
- Identify and engage someone in each child's life (in either the family or the larger community) who sees the child as important and who will maintain an active advocacy role for him or her.
- Offer an understanding of the limitations and difficulties of court-mandated treatment, and make attempts to restore a sense of control to parents/caretakers who may feel disempowered and overwhelmed by agency expectations.
- Finally, employ a team approach in which the limits of confidentiality are clearly understood by family members.

GOALS OF INTEGRATED TREATMENT

My goals are generally consistent with those of other professionals who specialize in the treatment of abused and traumatized children. Where they may differ is primarily in the integrated practice responses I recommend providing to children and their families. A pivotal aspect of treatment for abused and traumatized children is abuse-focused psychotherapy. As Karp and Butler (1996) put it, "the child's work is to gain the courage to go back to the frightening thoughts and images of the trauma and explore them in a safer environment when there is a better sense of control. The child must then gain the skills necessary to cope with what may be seen as a frightening world in which to grow up as a healthier adult" (p. xxiii). I concur with their subsequent statement that "the therapist's job is to create an environment in which the child can do this important work in a safe, nurturing, and protective setting" (p. xxiii).

These concepts and others have helped me to formulate the following goals of treatment for traumatized children:

- Develop a therapy relationship of mutual trust and respect.
- Help children identify their idiosyncratic perceptions, thoughts, feelings, and behaviors, with emphasis on their phenomenological experiences or attributions (Cohen & Mannarino, 2002).
- Help children with expression and externalization of important thoughts and feelings, utilizing a range of verbal and nonverbal engagement strategies (specified in Chapters Two, Four, and Five).
- Help children manage and regulate the expression of affect and behavior.
- Help children understand and broaden their self-definition, self-regard, and feelings of competence.
- Bring specific trauma memories into conscious awareness through a combination of directive and nondirective approaches, including verbal communication and narrating, as well as symbolic expression and posttraumatic play.
- Actively encourage integration of memories and creation of verbal or nonverbal narratives of the trauma, which might include expanded coping and adaptive processing.
- Encourage and allow children to release energy and affect through symbolic expression.
- Process the experience of trauma within a family context, so that secrecy and denial are broken, supportive relationships are developed or strengthened, family roles are discussed, and control is reestablished.

These therapy goals can be advanced in a variety of formats, including individual child therapy, group therapy, family therapy, specific parent–child therapies, and parent support groups. I discuss these formats next.

POSSIBLE THERAPY FORMATS
WITHIN AN INTEGRATED APPROACH

Individual Child Therapy

Individual child therapy can include traditional verbal psychotherapy (see, e.g., Reisman & Ribordy, 1993), expressive therapies (discussed in

Chapter Four), and CBT (discussed in Chapter Five). (It should be noted that versions of CBT specifically for sexually abused children are among the few forms of therapy for this population that can be described as "evidence-based.") Child therapy has evolved from isolated treatment to a more holistic approach in which the child's ecosystem is not only taken into account, but accessed and engaged (O'Connor, 1997; Stern, 2002). Generally speaking, the goals of individual therapy with abused children include clinical efforts to assess problem areas and resiliency, restore preabuse functioning, and ensure that children receive the guidance and support they need from family members who have had a chance to process their crisis responses. Clinicians maintain a special interest in trauma and its recovery, as well as issues related to the short- and long-term effects of child maltreatment. Because of this, abused children may be seen on a continuing basis, responding to their developmental changes and cognitive reevaluations of their earlier experience.

Group Therapy

Structured, Short-Term Groups

Structured, short-term, goal-specific group therapy has proven helpful for sexually abused children. These groups usually provide their members with immediate and concrete benefits: Sexually abused children can rapidly verify that their experience is not unique by meeting other sexually abused children. This produces relief and breaks their sense of isolation and stigmatization. In addition, sexually abused children can see and hear that other such children have worries and concerns similar to their own. For example, when group leaders assist children in talking about why they think sexual abuse happens, who it happens to, why grownups or older children abuse young children, or how children feel afterward, they realize very quickly that their reactions are not strange or bizarre. The fact that they can understand and relate to each other provides immeasurable assistance to these children, and it is possible that they can begin to normalize their reactions—to feel less "crazy" or "weird." It is important to note that such feelings, if unchallenged, can become rigid belief systems over time. Children need to understand the reality of events that occurred as soon as possible, to avoid the creation of or subsequent reliance on cognitive distortions.

Group therapy is almost always considered helpful for children. However, there are a few situations that could lessen a group's effectiveness. First, if children are experiencing acute PTSD, exposure to information from group members about their abuse might be overstimulating and contribute to deterioration. Second, if children are currently in court proceedings, their attendance at group and subsequent exposure to information about other children's situations could be considered contaminating. Third, when it's not certain whether abuse has actually occurred, children might benefit from group therapy that is less specific to child sexual abuse—for example, groups that target specific behavioral problems, such as anger or poor social skills. Finally, there are some children whose behavior is so dysregulated that they are not able to manage cooperative participation in group therapy and should continue in individual therapy to address affective and behavioral regulation. Several texts have been written to guide practitioners in setting up and designing structured group therapy for sexually abused children (Corder, 2000; Grotsky, Camerer, & Damiano, 2000). In addition, a website has been set up to disseminate information on setting up trauma-focused cognitive-behavioral groups (www. musc.edu/tfcbt).

Groups for Sexually Reactive Children

Sexually abused children struggle with many concerns and confusions, not the least of which are issues about sexuality. They may become either sexually preoccupied or sexually avoidant. In particular, sexual abuse seems to contribute to the emergence of sexualized behaviors and aggression (Berliner & Briere, 1997; Friedrich, 1990; Gallo-Lopez, 2005; McLeer, Deblinger, Henry, & Orvaschel, 1992). Problematic sexual behaviors may include excessive masturbation, masturbating in public, making verbally explicit and offensive comments and requests, and drawing sexually explicit images. These behaviors elicit negative responses from others and may cause a threat to peers who are exposed to inappropriate behaviors, language, and/or information. These children appear to be sexually overstimulated and may have made negative associations between sex and aggression or between sex and power/control. They need very specific guidance to correct and replace their problem behaviors, and they need to have ways of calming their anxious or impulsive feelings. Group therapy for sexually reactive children is behaviorally based and presents children with lesson plans, homework, and parental monitoring (see Gil & Johnson, 1993).

Children with sexual behavior problems are referred for therapy with greater frequency, and treatment resources for them are woefully absent. This lack of resources is a particular problem, since many programs for child *victims* will not provide services to young *victimizers*; this appears to be a gross oversight, since many abused children signal their victimization through sexual aggression. At present, groups for sexually reactive children are among the very few therapeutic options for such youngsters.

Family Therapy

Family therapy is essential work in cases of child abuse and can be provided at different intervals in therapy and at different levels (see Chapter Six for a full discussion). Stern (2002) eloquently describes something I myself learned early in my clinical work:

> I discovered that everything I knew and learned had a place and was useful in a collaborative family-centered therapy: there was no need to leave behind the individual work with the child; child sessions have an important place; family inclusion and involvement certainly move the work along; there were ways to make the treatment child-friendly and playful, to highlight the child's voice, and to help children and families take treatment home. (p. xii)

Some family therapy programs maintain a systemic focus from the intake sessions onward, requiring the presence of all family members throughout the therapy process. It is obvious that all family members are affected when child abuse occurs, and parents or caretakers often have parallel feelings of denial, secrecy, shock, confusion, anger, helplessness, and so forth. However, in my experience, a *child-focused* family therapy approach allows clinicians to assess and respond best to children's specific needs. Parents are engaged from the beginning of treatment to provide clinicians with relevant information about their children. Throughout the therapy process, parental needs are assessed, referrals are made as necessary, and family members are coached to respond appropriately and sensitively to the children. When family therapy sessions are provided, these have very specific goals.

For the most part, my experience has shown me that most parents or other caretakers who discover their children's abuse take the necessary steps to reconstruct a safe and nurturing environment, even if their initial reactions include varying levels of denial. However, I have also encountered some families in which parents/caretakers (particularly nonoffending mothers) seem to turn against their children and become punitive toward them for disclosing. In these cases, denial in all its forms (including minimization and rationalization) may persist; attempts to engage them in therapy fail; or they refuse to put the children's interest above other family interests (such as marital or financial stability). Some mothers cannot visualize their own ability to be self-sufficient; are untrained, unskilled, or unfamiliar with working outside the home; or may be emotionally dependent and reliant on the current family structure. In many such cases, mothers are forced to make fear-based decisions that they regret. It is often useful for mothers to attend support groups in which they can meet other mothers in similar situations and give and receive support, sometimes gaining the strength to make decisions that support their children. (See "Parent Support Groups," below.)

Psychopharmacology

I maintain a conservative view of medication for young children. However, some severely abused children may experience acute and debilitating symptoms that can be alleviated by use of medication, or that may require hospitalization or other higher levels of care. If psychopharmacology is indicated, nonprescribing clinicians must maintain active collaborative communication with treating physicians and must consistently review and document children's medications, children's reports of effects and outcomes, parents'/caretakers' willingness and ability to provide medications consistently, and parents'/caretakers' observation of medication effects and outcomes.

Specific Parent–Child Therapies

Filial Therapy

Filial therapy (Guerney, 1997, 2003; Van Fleet, 1994) is an evidence-based structured approach to restoring and enhancing parent–child relationships. It has been found to improve emotional connectedness, communication, and conflict negotiation. Parents are taught to conduct play sessions with their children; client-centered (Rogerian) approaches are used to help parents understand their children, respect their perspectives, and provide appropriate limits. This approach designates the parents, under the supervision and instruction of an experienced play therapist, as the primary change agents for their children. A specific didactic component that incorporates learning theory and behavioral principles is an integral part of the structured play sessions. Parents who utilize filial therapy well communicate a respectful attitude to their children, whose sense of self increases. Guerney (1997) speculates that as children experience their parents in the role of the therapist, they and their parents will feel more positive toward each other, and thus their relationships will improve. This approach has been shown to be effective in altering inappropriate or ineffective parenting behaviors in a variety of settings.

Parent–Child Interaction Therapy

Parent–child interaction therapy (PCIT) is another evidence-based therapy for enhancing parent–child relationships. It was developed by Sheila Eyberg (Eyberg, 1988; Hembree-Kigin & McNeill, 1995) and has been effectively used for families with child abuse problems (Borrego, Urquiza, Rasmussen, & Zebell, 1999). PCIT provides highly specified, step-by-step, live-coached sessions with both a parent/caregiver alone and the adult and child together. The parent/caregiver learns skills through PCIT didactic sessions, and then is coached in specific skills (via a transmitter-and-receiver system) as he or she interacts in specific play with the child. Generally the therapist provides the coaching from behind a one-way mirror, and the emphasis is on changing parent/caregiver–child patterns of interaction.

Parent Support Groups

It is important to provide support and guidance to parents/caretakers who discover that their children have been sexually abused. (Historically, the vast majority of individuals committing sexual offenses have been male, and in cases of intrafamilial sexual abuse the offenders are most often fathers or stepfathers. Based on these facts, professionals in the field of child sexual abuse identification and treatment often describe parent support groups as being for "nonoffending parents" or specifically for "nonoffending mothers.") Support groups can be either psychoeducational or purely supportive. Both types of groups allow parents/caretakers to meet others going through the same experience. In addition, psychoeducational groups provide specific information, including definitions of abuse, incidence, types of offenses, reasons why offenders molest children, family dynamics, and short- and long-term consequences. Parents are also instructed about the helping team of professionals, multiple agency roles, and processes that may be underway in the legal and/or child welfare systems. Parents often find that broadening their knowledge base about sexual abuse is empowering and helps them to make or maintain important decisions and choices about their families' needs, safety, and general functioning.

SUMMARY

There is general agreement about the psychological, emotional, and behavioral consequences of child maltreatment, especially sexual abuse. In addition, recent research has confirmed that trauma causes alterations in children's neurological development. This more comprehensive view of effects should guide clinicians in selecting their interventions and tailoring them to individual children's needs.

To date, there have been few treatment outcome studies with populations of traumatized children; however, as interest grows in identifying evidence-based clinical practices, practitioners are encouraged to find ways to incorporate research strategies into their clinical practices. A few therapies have been the objects of such study, and their effectiveness has been demonstrated (e.g., CBT techniques; see Chapter Five), while other methods have not yet gathered sufficient scientific support. It's important to note that validation of one technique does not automatically invalidate others. Traditionally, psychotherapists have utilized strategies that are well grounded in theory and that appear to have positive results for their clients. Strategies that either include or exclude families have been utilized by child therapists. In addition, contemporary child therapists value an interactive role with children's larger systems, especially schools.

Clinicians in private practice may not have the ability (or willingness) to construct research projects that validate their work, but they often utilize goal attainment scaling (Justice & Justice, 1979) or other methods of defining, reviewing, and achieving their stated goals. Meeting stated goals might also demonstrate the effectiveness of diverse approaches. It is important to note that several studies of therapy's effectiveness in general point to clients' perception of therapists' warmth; that is, clients seem to make progress when they like and feel liked by their therapists (Miller, Duncan, & Hubble, 1997).

CBT approaches are currently at the forefront of empirically based treatment. However, it's important to note that the literature in the field of child sexual abuse repeatedly emphasizes that children have difficulty articulating their abuse or addressing it directly. In addition to children's natural resistance to talking about the abuse due to shame, guilt, fear, or lack of awareness that abuse is inappropriate, evidence also suggests that trauma memories are imbedded in the right hemisphere of the brain, and thus that interventions facilitating access to and activity in the right side of the brain may be indicated. The right hemisphere of the brain is most receptive to nonverbal strategies that utilize symbolic language, creativity, and pretend play. Thus art, play, sand, and other expressive therapies may be necessary components of trauma treatment.

It is also clear that no two abused or traumatized children are alike, and that there is no rigid, unvarying profile of such children. Therefore children will enter therapy with a wide range of emotional and behavioral problems as well as defensive strategies. In addition, child therapists need to attend to differences resulting from culture, gender, and developmental age and stage. Because of all these variables, clinicians need to remain flexible, interested, and responsive to each child's unique needs.

The rest of this text unfolds an integrated treatment approach that recognizes and values different therapeutic perspectives, and utilizes them in a purposeful and discriminating manner.

4

Expressive Therapies

$\mathbf{P}$roviding therapy to young children and adolescents requires clinicians to engage with them at their individual developmental levels and to invite their participation in creative and compelling ways. When clinicians work with abused and traumatized children, they cannot rely too heavily on any specific approach or on children's willingness to use verbal communication; rather, they need to have a broad range of both verbal and nonverbal techniques at their disposal. "Expressive therapies" is a term used to define the therapeutic use of the arts and play with children and adults individually, in groups, or in family sessions. The media used in expressive therapies include many different visual/manual arts and crafts, music, dance/movement, drama, play, writing (poetry and journaling), and sandplay and other sand therapies. McNiff (cited in Malchiodi, 2005), who founded the first Expressive Therapies Graduate Program at Lesley University in 1974, states, "these therapies have been used since ancient times as preventative and reparative forms of treatment. There are numerous references within medicine, anthropology, and the arts to the earliest healing applications of expressive modalities" (p. 4). We are fortunate that McNiff and many others have paved the way toward greater understanding and applicability of expressive therapies, which can be used as primary or adjunctive approaches, depending on a clinician's level of training and experience with them. This chapter highlights three specific expressive therapies that I have found useful with abused and traumatized children (i.e., play, art, and sand therapies), but I encourage readers to think of all such therapies as potentially useful.

ORIGINS AND DEVELOPMENT
OF THREE EXPRESSIVE THERAPIES

Three creative, distinctive, and inspired methods for child and adult therapy were developed within the same approximate time period; were crafted for similar purposes by professional women; and have had parallel outcomes, impact, and longevity. Art therapy, play therapy, and sand therapy were advanced by psychoanalysts as innovative approaches that would help both child and adult clients externalize and manage their internal worlds, and these therapies are currently viewed as highly relevant and practical for work with children.

Art Therapy

Rubin (1987) notes that Sigmund Freud, in developing his psychoanalytic theory, recognized early that patients used expressive techniques and that their "most important communications were descriptions of visual images" (p. 7). Clearly, Freud's interest in his patients' dreams was an attempt to elicit the translation of images into words. Rubin notes that Freud would often "actively request images" (p. 7), by instructing his clients to concentrate on forgotten memories or by placing his hand on their foreheads so they could feel external pressure. Freud later abandoned this interest in visual images for a process he labeled "free association" (the process of verbalizing free-process thinking). Anna Freud, his daughter and herself a child psychoanalyst, renewed the focus on art (as well as play), because she found that her young child patients were not well suited to make use of the process of free association.

Beginning in the late 1940s, Margaret Naumburg facilitated the integration of Freudian insights about "unconscious communication through imagery and the use of art therapy" (Rubin, 1987, p. 9). Naumburg called her approach "dynamically oriented art psychotherapy" and viewed it as serving the function of a "primary therapeutic method," rather than as an "auxiliary to other forms of treatment" (Ulman, Kramer, & Kwiatkowska, 1977, p. 7). About a decade later (in the late 1950s), Edith Kramer, also a psychoanalyst, began developing a view of art therapy as complementary to psychotherapy—"bringing unconscious material closer to the surface," and "providing an area of symbolic experience wherein changes may be tried out" (Ulman et al., 1977, p. 8).

Elinor Ulman, yet another art therapy pioneer, brought the two views offered by Naumburg and Kramer together, suggesting that art therapy covers "a broad range of endeavors limited only by the requirement that they must genuinely partake of both art and therapy" (Ulman et al., 1977, p. 9). Slowly, art as a means to advance therapeutic goals became a credible resource to those who were both formally trained and/or untrained in the arts. Recent efforts have been made by Malchiodi (1998) and others (Furth, 2002; Oster & Montgomery, 1996) to bridge the gap in knowledge between specially trained art therapists and those child therapists who routinely use art activities in their clinical practices without the benefit of formal training. Recognizing that formal art therapy training may not be desirable or possible for many therapists who work with children, and that for some therapists art will never become a central therapeutic approach, Malchiodi (1998) in particular provides a comprehensive foundation that encourages more responsible utilization of art work with children—although she also emphasizes the necessity to obtain additional training and consultation in this area. In a subsequent edited text, Malchiodi (2003) once again highlights the value and power of art therapy in different settings, with different populations, and within differing treatment modalities. The usefulness of art therapy continues to be documented for different populations, and several publications describe the use of art therapy for individuals with histories of sexual abuse (Gil, 2003a; Gerity, 1999; Brooke, 1995; Cohen, Barnes, & Rankin, 1995; Cohen & Cox, 1995).

Play Therapy

It is difficult to imagine a time when children were not seen as viable candidates for therapy; however, up until Freud's first documented efforts to help a child, most analysts would only venture into the mental health treatment of adults. Due to Freud's significant influence on the clinical community, his first therapeutic success with a child's symptoms of phobia (Freud, 1909/1955) laid the foundation for later work with children. Whereas Hug-Hellmuth (1921) used play more directly with children in their own homes, believing that it was an essential part of child analysis, Anna Freud and Melanie Klein have long been regarded as the predominant forces behind the use of play with children in therapy.

Anna Freud (1965) initially viewed play as a way to lure children into therapy and to establish a therapeutic alliance between a clinician and a child patient with the goal of achieving transference responses in the child. She elicited verbalizations from children as soon as they became more comfortable with her through the use of toys and games, and once she solidified the alliance. Melanie Klein (1932), however, was much more interested in using play as a direct substitute for verbalizations (equivalent to the free associations of adult patients). She considered play a child's natural mechanism for expression and communication. Accordingly, Klein (1932) treated play activities as "primary data on which to base interpretations" (p. 11). These two pioneers viewed play interpretations as potentially therapeutic, but differed on the amount of interpreting that was necessary or useful. Esman (1983) notes that "the dominant influence in child analytic practice in the United States has been Anna Freud, her pupils, and her associates, and it is, by and large, her approach that has dominated the theory and practice of play therapy in clinical work with children in this country" (p. 12).

O'Connor (1991) suggests that the major therapeutic goal of psychoanalytic play is the "development or revision of psychic structures and functions" (p. 18), so that optimal development can occur. This is done through interpretation and working through of art or play, which may promote the child's insight and behavioral change. Psychoanalytic play therapy has serious limitations, however, because it is recommended for those children who have clearly developed personalities and whose "symptoms arise from anxiety produced by internal conflict" (O'Connor, 1991, p. 18). This type of therapy is viewed as most effective for clients who can verbalize, gain insights, and then implement behavioral changes.

Others have expanded the use of psychoanalytic play therapy. Levy (1939) developed a play therapy model called "release therapy," based on the psychoanalytic concept of the benefit of repetition compulsion. Levy's therapeutic model was most suitable to children who had experienced traumatic events and who could assimilate negative thoughts and feelings through play reenactments of the traumatic material. This model is the foundation for contemporary thinking on the value and usefulness of posttraumatic play (Terr, 1983, 1990), which I discuss in greater detail in Chapter Seven.

Since the early development of psychoanalytic play therapy, other major play therapy models have emerged—most notably behavioral (Skinner, 1972; Bandura, 1977), cognitive-behavioral (Knell, 1993), developmental (Brody, 1978, 1993; Jernberg, 1979), ecosystemic (O'Connor, 1994), Gestalt (Oaklander, 1988, 1994), humanistic (Rogers, 1951; Axline, 1947; Moustakas, 1959; Landreth, 1982; Rank, 1936), and Adlerian (Kottman, 1995). O'Connor (1991) notes that these theories share a basic respect for the various functions of play. These include biological development (skill building), intrapersonal development (fulfillment of both the human need to do something and the drive for mastery), and interpersonal development (achievement of individuation/separation from the primary caretaker, as well as acquisition of social skills). Through all three of these functions, play therapy embodies curative factors that can benefit children and adults alike (Schaefer, 1993). Amster (1982) notes that in the transition from play as play to play as therapy, several uses have been well established: to increase diagnostic understanding; to establish a working relationship; to break through a child's defenses; to facilitate communication and verbalization; to help the child act out unconscious material and to release accompanying tension; and to promote developmental growth.

It is interesting to note that although art therapy, play therapy, and (as will be documented below) sand therapy all had their origins in psychoanalytic theory and were first developed within the same time period (the early 1900s), the developers of each type of therapy took little interest in the work of the others, and few if any exchanges took place among them. As a result, these models and approaches, now conventional tools of child therapy, evolved in relative isolation from each other.

Sand Therapy

In 1911, the British novelist and political writer H. G. Wells chronicled his work with children in a book entitled *Floor Games* (an American edition has been republished; Wells, 1911/1975). Wells and his two sons engaged in elaborate floor games, including, for example, the building of cities; they used miniatures of people and animals, and construction materials that included wood, paper, and plasticine. Margaret Lowenfeld, who read the book when she was about 21 years old, was fascinated with the description of this play and integrated this type of work with children into her later analytic practice. Lowenfeld was a practicing pediatrician for a number of years and left that profession to become a child psychiatrist. She purchased the equipment Wells suggested and kept it in what her child clients called "the wonder box" (Lowenfeld, 1979, p. 3). In 1929, she added zinc trays to her basic equipment—one filled with sand, and the other with water. She stored her miniatures in a cabinet, and found that children quite naturally brought the miniatures to the sand trays and built scenarios in the sand, which she called "worlds." Bowyer (1970) notes that within a 3-month period, these children had in fact created a new technique; Lowenfeld's remarkable ability to follow, rather than lead, allowed this amazing process to take place. Lowenfeld eventually called this process the "world technique" (Lowenfeld, 1979). Thompson (1981/1990) notes that it has remained virtually unchanged since its beginning, and includes "imaginative activity with the sand, used with or without objects, within a circumscribed space, in the presence of a therapist" (p. 7).

Lowenfeld demonstrated the world technique at several international conferences as early as 1939. Dora Kalff, a Swiss Jungian child analyst, was immediately captivated and became one of Lowenfeld's best students, consulting as well with Carl Jung, her mentor throughout her career. Kalff inspired many Jungian analysts as she taught and lectured widely on the effectiveness of what she renamed "sandplay" (Kalff, 1980), and virtually introduced this method in the United States. Kalff's Jungian background has influenced many Jungian analysts to use sandplay; many people also associate sandplay with strict Jungian principles, which in some ways may have made this technique less accessible to the wider professional community. In fact, Spare (1981/1990) confides that her colleagues "often spoke to me of their intimidation at what they feel to be an exclusivity or even preciosity surrounding the use of the sand tray as a clinical instrument. . . . they express an intense sense of awe and wonder in which sandplay takes on something of the numinosity and power of an archetype of change" (p. 195).

Contemporary clinicians (Labovitz Boik & Goodwin, 2000; Carey, 1999; Dundas, 1978; Allan & Berry, 1987; Weinrib, 1983; De Domenico, 1988) continue to develop, present, and promote a range of expanded approaches to sand therapy. Mitchell and Friedman (1994) describe sandplay as one of the fastest-growing therapies. They aptly chronicle the past, present, and future directions of this therapeutic technique, highlighting and contrasting the contributions of the pioneers mentioned above, as well as others (e.g., Bühler, 1951) who have had an impact on professional interest and research in this approach.

Most proponents of Jungian-based sandplay agree that this process engages the active imaginative or creative process, promotes a developmental or healing process, externalizes the client's internal world, serves as an impetus for release of psychic energy, and is essentially a process that can often bridge conscious and unconscious processes. As such, a therapist is encouraged to say little throughout a client's sand therapy process, and to be cautious about interpreting what is seen. As Weinrib (1983) points out, "the specific interpretation of a particular symbol may be less important than the process itself and the relationship between [the therapist] and the client" (p. 16). Weinrib adds that "sandplay brings to the therapeutic process the element of genuinely free play, with all that it implies in terms of freedom and creativity. Sandplay is not a game with rules. It is free and encourages playfulness. Its value lies in its experiential noncerebral character" (p. 17). Although there are few specific rules per se (see Spare, 1981/1990), Weinrib notes eight basic concepts that guide the use of sandplay:

1. Psychological development, under normal circumstances, is similar for everyone.
2. The psyche consists of consciousness and unconsciousness and the interaction between them, and contains a drive toward wholeness and a tendency to heal itself.
3. The self is the totality of the personality and its directing center.
4. The unconscious is the source of psychological life in the same way that the mother is the source of physical life. The mother and

the unconscious therefore can be seen as symbolic feminine equivalents, with the drive to return to the mother as the drive to the return to the unconscious.

5. Psychological healing involves restoration of the capacity to function normally, whereas ego-consciousness relates to awareness and choice of what we are doing while we function.

6. Psychological healing is an emotional, nonrational phenomenon that takes place at the preverbal level.

7. Both healing and expansion of consciousness are desirable ends in psychotherapy.

8. The natural healing process can effectively be activated by therapeutic play and stimulation of creative impulses via conditions provided in the tray.

Weinrib also emphasizes the necessity and value of the free and protected space that using the sand tray clearly provides.[1]

As the descriptions above indicate, art, play, and sand therapies can provide a clinician with astounding access to an individual's unconscious material, and the therapist's responses and engagement with the client can either enhance or dilute the client's creative process and product. Training in these specialized fields of study is therefore not only desirable, but necessary, to maximize the potential to help and minimize the potential for damage. An unforgettable book, written by a therapist who herself had a nervous breakdown resulting in part from her work with an injured child, candidly chronicles both the harmful and the healing possibilities of psychotherapy (Rogers, 1995).

These three distinct expressive therapies have their foundations in psychoanalytic theory, as noted above. They seek to engage the unconscious, glean conflicts or concerns, and promote insight, which then is viewed as a means to achieve beneficial behavioral changes. They have all been used effectively in educational and health arenas to stimulate, promote, or optimize developmental and reparative processes.

These three approaches, when used by trained professionals, have

---

[1] As sand therapy has gained popularity, clinicians have improvised in an effort to stock the necessary equipment at reasonable cost. Some clinicians use kitty litter boxes or Tupperware boxes as sand trays. It is important to note that Lowenfeld (1979) proposed the dimensions for a sand tray as 50 x 75 centimeters. Kalff (1980) proposed the dimensions of 19.5 x 28.5 x 3 inches. Kalff in particular discussed the importance of comfort for sand builders: The builder should be able to look at the entire tray without moving the head, and to reach all corners of the tray comfortably. She also recommended that the tray be waist-high to the user, and that trays of different heights be used whenever possible.

the capacity to facilitate a wide variety of individual strategies (e.g., withdrawal or expansion, camouflage or disclosure, integration or compartmentalization, structuring or unmassing of psychological mechanisms) that may assist in a healing outcome. In addition, all three therapies can hasten engagement with the unconscious, in that they provide kinetic, sensory, and physical experiences—they can be felt, smelled, touched, tasted, and remembered. The clinical opportunities are promising when these approaches are used independently, and awesome when they are used in combination. In my experience, children can readily go from one therapeutic mode to another (either spontaneously or by suggestion), and the combination of these three therapy options can provide clinicians with cumulative diagnostic or prognostic information. Using these three approaches interactively also appears to offer children (and sometimes adolescents and adults as well) increased reparative opportunities. The images and metaphors provided by children in one type of therapy can be amplified, enriched, made more tangible, and developed to a greater extent in another, as I will show in the clinical illustrations in the second part of this book.

SIMILARITIES/DIFFERENCES AMONG ART, PLAY, AND SAND THERAPIES

Art, play, and sand therapies have common characteristics as well as unique attributes. First and foremost, all three are universal activities that children experience throughout the developmental process, to one degree or another. Parents may promote, inspire, or facilitate their children's creativity or imagination—or, conversely, may diminish or obstruct their desire for these forms of expression. Parents seem to value self-expression through objects or symbols at varying levels of interest. For example, some parents refuse to purchase or provide formal toys for children, preferring to encourage children either to transform generic objects into play objects or to build toys for themselves.

Children themselves may use art, play, or sand therapy spontaneously or when directed to do so, and either frequently or intermittently. As they mature, they may replace these modes of communication or self-expression in favor of verbal communication and rational, concrete thinking. Adults often use their creativity and imagination minimally, making rigid separations between adult and child activities or behaviors.

Moreover, because art, play, and sandplay are familiar, user-friendly activities to children, they can engage easily with these techniques. Children tend to feel reassured as they enter therapy offices and see some of the objects (e.g., crayons and paper, miniature cars) that signal the possibility of known, pleasurable activities. They make swift, positive associations that help to put them at ease, and that may make the owner of the objects (i.e., the therapist) less ominous or distant.

Finally, art, play, and sandplay are transformed in a clinical setting, because there is a clinical goal and an observer who makes efforts to understand, decode, and provide helpful clinical responses. By definition, a therapist who uses one or more of these approaches is also creating a safe, structured, accepting environment in which a child may eventually reveal secrets, develop insight, adapt to circumstances, improve coping strategies, and repair psychological damage. For children with emotional difficulties, these three therapies allow them to bring out hidden concerns, whether they intend to reveal them or not.

Art therapy materials provide young art makers with a range of options. Some children revel in the control they can exert with a finely sharpened pencil, creating shading of light to heavy intensity. Others prefer the freedom of splattering fluid paints on large canvases that seem to catch the paints, forming images that come alive and speak not only to their makers but to others. Still other clients find using fluid paints a regressive experience; they seem engrossed with the tactile experience of placing their fingers and hands in paints, making squishy noises, and making the paints more liquid or solid. The process of art making involves the senses to differing degrees, and art makers comment on the diverse smells, feel, sound, and look of chosen media. Obviously, the materials an individual chooses to use to make art, or the materials that are made available, advocated, or avoided by the art therapist, may either hasten or obstruct contact with a range of feelings and reactions. Consequently, the art therapist and art maker alike must remain sensitive and alert to the art maker's process and potential benefits or disadvantages of using one medium or another. Art making can be done on small or large pieces of paper, on construction paper, or on formal canvases. More modern, abstract art can also be created on a variety of surfaces and materials (e.g., wall murals on buildings brighten up many cities). But the most traditional use of art is on paper, and paper of any size (or color) has edges that serve as boundaries. The art maker always reacts to a contained space, filling it as much or as little as he or she wants.

When someone completes an art process, a tangible product remains that can be either admired, appreciated, or disregarded. The art maker chooses whether to keep or discard the art, to hide it or display it openly. Once a product is created, the art maker also has the option to *see* or *not to see* the meaning of images he or she has created. Moreover, the maker decides who will see an art product and what will be told about it. Many decisions must be made once the product is complete. Some art makers leave their products behind without a second glance, may abruptly destroy what has been made, may direct the art therapist to keep the products for them, or may want to take them home for safekeeping. The product may also produce positive, negative, or neutral feelings in the art maker. Unfortunately, some makers focus on the product's representational qualities—that is, how much it looks like what they were trying to make. Often art makers feel that they fall short in their artistic abilities, and the art product becomes symbolic of their negative self-image. Sadly, some individuals won't even engage in art because of their feelings of performance anxiety. Some can be swayed from their expectations of artistic perfection by instruction in abstract art making; others resist abstract art, finding the images disturbing and unexplainable.

When resistance to making art cannot be overcome, I suggest making art in a sand tray. As a matter of fact, some clinicians routinely ask clients to make "pictures" in sand, rather than asking them to make "worlds" in sand. In sand therapy, the individual is not expected to make representational images, but rather to use miniatures (which are provided) to create a scenario. Individuals are asked to create whatever they want, using as few or as many miniatures as they wish. The boundaries provided by the edges of paper in art therapy are made concrete by the substantial and visible walls of a sand tray in sand therapy.

Although the art maker who uses paper chooses the size of paper he or she wishes to use on any given day, the sand therapy client will be limited by the standard size of the traditional sand tray. The worlds that are created in sand are therefore created within the same dimensions each time, although children's creativity can never be underestimated. Although almost always adults stay within the boundaries of one tray, children may build bridges to other trays, or somehow link up the world in the sand to other play materials. One child with whom I worked moved a sand tray next to the dollhouse and made a path leading from the front of the house to the "beach," using the entire sand tray to make an ocean scene within walking distance for the family that lived in the dollhouse.

Sand therapy, like art, also provides opportunities for fluid or resistive activity, since water can be poured into sand trays; this allows the makers of sand worlds to shape, amass, mold, flood, or otherwise experience wet sand. Depending on the amount of water used, sand will respond differently.

The products that are created in sand trays are not permanent, since the trays are inevitably dismantled and prepared for future use. A sand world can be chronicled, however, by taking a photograph that captures the scenario created on any given day. Unfortunately, a photo does not always capture idiosyncratic detail; also, depending on the angle at which the photo is taken, one or another aspect may be emphasized, providing a less than accurate or full view of the world. Nevertheless, the photo does provide a hint of what was created, and it allows the client an opportunity to recreate a product, pursue a theme, or simply create a new, unrelated product.

Play therapy is yet another powerful avenue for self-expression, communication, and self-soothing. Objects (toys, miniatures) are provided to the child, although children possess the ability to use imagination and fantasy to assign various meanings to each object. For example, a Popsicle stick that has just been used as a pretend gun to kill someone can immediately be transformed into a tongue depressor to medically assist the person who's been shot and revived.

Play will be used by children in representational or abstract form, depending on their age. A child goes through stages of play, much in the same way that art appears to have specific qualities, depending on the child's age and cognitive ability (Lowenfeld & Brittain, 1987). Play also has specific stages that reflect children's growth (Schaefer, Gitlin, & Sandgrund, 1991); as such, both play and art can be used for developmental assessment as well as for specific diagnostic and treatment purposes.

Play does not have the concrete boundaries offered by art and sand therapies. Children can create stories, undo them, transform them, forget them, or keep bringing them up. Once toys are used, they are put back, and the next time they may be ignored or may be assigned completely different meanings.

Children may use all three of these distinctive therapies in an absorbed, focused way, being extremely involved with their own process and screening out the environment. Or they may interact with the clinician throughout the whole process—asking for approval, attention, or direction; wanting the clinician to participate in the product development or play; assigning or taking roles; giving voices to characters; or responding to questions posed by the clinician.

THE USE OF SPECIFIC EXPRESSIVE TECHNIQUES
IN ASSESSMENT AND TREATMENT

No matter what type of expressive therapy is used, a clinician is able to gather important information about a child by observing and documenting two dimensions: the *process* of the art, play, or sand therapy, and the *content* (of the product) presented. The process informs the clinician about the child's affective engagement with the materials (tone, posture, activity level, approach–avoidance, absorption, and physical involvement are observed). The content is the symbol, metaphor, or story presented through the use of the materials (organization and style, repetition, presence of conflict and resolution, and possible links to real-life issues). Both process and content can provide significant data in the course of assessment (particularly the extended developmental assessment described in Chapter Two) and treatment. I have found in the course of my own work that certain expressive techniques yield particularly valuable information about children's perceptions of their life situations, relationships, worries, or joys; I describe these techniques below.

Play Genograms

As described in the case example of Gene in Chapter Two, children can be asked to provide play genograms. First, a clinician and child construct a genogram on a large piece of easel paper. Genogram construction can take one or a few sessions, depending on children's interest in and knowledge about their families. Some genograms can include birth, foster, or adoptive families; friends and pets; teachers; healthcare professionals; and other caretakers. The addition of friends, pets, and "other important people in your life" may actually provide a significant mapping of children's external resources—that is, the people they regard as important in their lives. Often extended family members, teachers, day care providers, or social workers may be major sources of support, warmth, or guidance to children. Finding out about "forgotten" or marginalized family members can also be informative.

Once a play genogram is completed, and all important people are included visually, two distinct instructions can be given to increase its value. The first instruction is to "choose a miniature that best shows your thoughts and feelings about each person in your family, including yourself." Children are told to pick the miniatures and place them on the circles or squares that represent family members on the genogram. The instructions do not emphasize a limit on the number of miniatures, so it is informative to watch children negotiate the need for additional miniatures, to show a wider range of thoughts or feelings about specific family members or friends.

Children approach this first task in a variety of ways. Recently a teenager seemed actively resistant to undertaking this task, and I commended her on how well she had explained her reluctance to use expressive techniques (this reluctance to use expressive techniques coincided with her unwillingness to communicate verbally). Finally she acquiesced to the task, and I opted to take a bathroom break so that she wouldn't feel self-conscious about starting the play genogram. She was so absorbed in the task that she did not hear me open the door and reenter the room, and she seemed oblivious to my presence for at least the next 10 minutes. When she looked up and told me she was "done," she had selected and used the most amazing array of miniatures, incredibly rich in symbolism (see Figure 4.1). In spite of her initial protests, this youngster was very adept at completing this task in a way that allowed her to present new information.

As Figure 4.1 shows, this girl, Heidi, used the figure of an alien to describe herself and her internal experience of feeling isolated, different, and disconnected from others. The alien figure stood alone but was also quite central, while facing forward and turning her back to all the miniatures behind her. It was almost as if her family existed separately from her (something she verbalized when she began to talk about the play genogram). I asked this teen to tell me about the alien, and she noted, "That alien feels completely alone, weird—like everyone stares at her, doesn't understand her, and won't even give her a chance." I wondered aloud about the alien's feelings and what the alien did with these feelings. "Mostly keep them to herself . . . she speaks in a different language and no one really understands her." "And if someone could understand her," I asked, "what would become obvious?" "How much she wants to have a friend." This girl was able to talk about her true feelings as long as we were talking about the alien in front of us.

Heidi then told me about the miniatures she had chosen for her mother: a unicorn with wings, and a three-headed figure with six arms. She said, "I chose the Pegasus for my mother because she's always leaving. You never know when she's going to stay or go. And I chose the three-headed person because you never know which mother you're go-

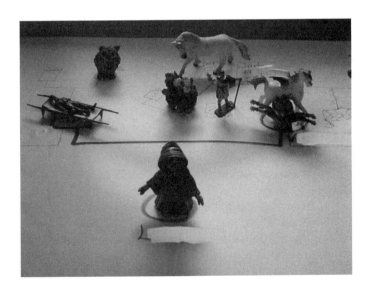

FIGURE 4.1. Heidi's play genogram.

ing to get. Often she has lots of different moods, and sometimes she gets kind of wild and chaotic, so I thought all the heads and arms kind of show that." This teen's most distressing issue was her mother's inability to maintain a firm, consistent relationship with her. We spent two sessions further identifying the difficulty in the mother–daughter relationship and discussing a realistic strategy to protect her from feeling constant disappointment.

Very young children can complete this project as well. It's best to ask for their participation, in order to determine their ability and/or willingness to cooperate. I have obtained play genograms from children as young as 5, and there is no maximum age limit. Adults tend to assert their surprise at how difficult it can be to choose miniatures—and, at the same time, how much they can learn from them. Children and adults alike vary in their choice of abstract or concrete symbols. For example, one 7-year-old boy picked a fireman because his father was a fireman; an 8-year-old girl chose a chicken because her mother liked to eat fried chicken; a 6-year-old selected a car because his dad was a mechanic. At the other end of the continuum, a 7-year-old girl picked out a sun for her grandmother because she was always smiling and nice to everyone; a teenage boy picked out a broken ship, insisting that he felt he was sinking; a 12-year-old boy picked out a scream figure for his mother, describing her as "holding a lot in, but really being unhappy and frustrated."

Two of my all-time favorite symbolic figures were chosen by a teenage girl and a frustrated mother, respectively. The teenager could not find the right symbol for her mother and finally constructed one out of clay, making first a square box, and then a head with nose, eyes, ears, and a big open mouth. Next she asked me for a ballpoint pen (I had one, luckily), and she took it apart, using the small spring inside to put between the box and the head. "This is my mom," she said with a glint in her eye, "Jack in the Box . . . she's wound up tightly, and you never know when she's going to blow." This gave us great opportunities for further discussion. The second memorable symbol use was when a very frustrated mother used a fire hydrant to express her perception that her family was in constant crisis and that she always had to "put out fires."

The play genogram can be used in only this first way with children, adolescents, and adults, or can be further amplified to include information about children's relational perceptions. The second instruction that can be given is this: "Pick a miniature that best shows your thoughts and feelings about the relationship you have with each person in your family, and put these miniatures between yourself and the other person." Because it can take a couple of sessions to construct the genogram and then select and place the miniatures on easel paper, the "relationship" activity is best done in one full session. The use of photographs to chronicle play genograms will allow individuals to recreate the original play genograms on their easel pages, which are carefully stored in art folders. This second play genogram activity is quite revealing. One adolescent put a small brick wall between himself and his father, noting, "I feel that I can't get through. You're like a wall and you don't give." At the same time, the father was touched by the fact that the wall chosen by his son was the smaller of two brick walls: "Well, at least this wall won't be as hard to tear down as the other one." I was impressed that this teen's father was able to accept the criticism and then convey some optimism about change.

In conjoint family sessions, all family members are given essentially the same first instruction described above: "Choose a miniature that best shows your thoughts and feelings about each person in the family, including yourself." They are then guided to explore the shelves with miniatures, and to take their time, explore, and ask if there's something they can't find.[2] Miniatures are then placed on the boxes and squares on the large piece of easel paper, and even the act of accommodating individual choices can be very indicative of family roles, alliances, collusions, and collective perceptions (Gil, 2003a).

There are no rigid or restrictive rules about how to conduct this task. The only caution I provide is that it does not seem to be productive to have each family member take an individual turn choosing miniatures. In my experience, turn-taking can contribute to individuals' feeling self-conscious, rushing selections, and looking for validation or other reactions from other family members before making choices. As a result, the task can become stymied and anxiety-provoking. It's best to allow all family members to get out of their chairs and peruse the miniatures at the same time, even though everyone choosing at the same time can also be a little difficult to track. In larger families, the selection process can generate a lot of dialogue, negotiation, fun, irritability, and challenge. The largest family group I worked with consisted of two parents, one grandparent, a former foster parent, and four young children. There were a minimum of 7 and a maximum of 13 miniatures on the easel paper. For the second task (inquiring about relationships), I drew the two genograms (for the birth and foster families) on an expanded piece of paper (two large pieces of easel paper taped together), and we moved to a room with a large oval desk on which the paper could be properly spread out. I offered each family member a small tray to collect his or her miniatures to be carried to the adjacent office.

After the miniatures are placed on the genogram, I make the follow-

---

[2] I keep soft, malleable plasticine in case someone is unable to find just what he or she wants and instead is willing to use clay to make the object.

ing request: "Now that you've placed your miniatures on the paper, I'd like you to look around, notice the miniatures that have been chosen, and talk a little together as a family. This is a time to show your interest, be curious, ask questions, make comments, and express anything you want about the miniatures you've placed on the paper." These dialogues usually bring a range of responses, including humor, insightfulness, defensiveness, interest, and concern. Every now and then negative feelings are expressed harshly, or several family members seem to gather strength from each other and complain about one other member. The family process is made explicit, and further discussion is elicited by clinical questions or directives.

There is an obvious need for family play genograms to be conducted by trained family therapists who can guide the family through difficult encounters and can maximize positive outcomes. My impression is that depending on the family therapist's particular orientation, the focus of the family work will take many shapes and forms. Someone interested in Gestalt therapy may ask family members to "be" the miniatures—that is, to give the miniatures voices. Narrative therapists may want to focus on expanding the range of chosen miniatures. Thus, if someone has picked a miniature that suggests anger in a family member, a narrative therapist may request an additional figure to express what the person is like when he or she is not angry. The possibilities are endless, and the family play genogram provides numerous opportunities for clearer communication, introspection, renewed family energy, and positive change.

Sand Therapy Activities: Following Clients' Leads

As described earlier, sand therapy in general is an appealing, low-difficulty task that most children and adults approach and engage with readily. Sand already has positive associations for many children, although children who have never visited a beach are likewise drawn to it. I have met a few rare individuals who withdraw from the feel of dry or wet sand, but touching and playing with sand can produce pleasurable physiological and emotional responses in most people, and clients almost always show or state their feelings of calm, relaxation, enjoyment, and delight.

Many children will respond positively to sand therapy when they seem reluctant to draw or paint. The unfortunate fear of not drawing well enough can be a powerful deterrent to children's or adults' enjoyment of art. In sand therapy, children are free simply to select from a broad range of objects, and somehow this decreases their anxiety about producing something that will be judged by others. Children may sometimes review their art products and lack confidence about what they've produced, but these feelings don't seem to play a major role in sand therapy.

Some children spend time playing with the sand in very primitive and relaxing ways: pushing the sand from one side to another, using a paintbrush to make shapes in the box, playing hide and seek with their hands, patting the sand with the palms of their hands, using their fingers to make circles or lines, filling and pouring cups, making hills or mountains, making lakes or rivers, or simply using a sifter to clean the sand. Other children make "worlds" in the sand almost immediately and can build underwater scenes, villages, fantasy lands, zoos, wild forests, spiritual places, their homes or rooms, and other environments. They may place miniatures to "protect" or "guard"; they may put down "bad" or "dangerous" animals or people; they may include parents and children in various forms; they may present themes of danger, safety, peace, activity, or industry.

During sand activities, I record children's thematic material, miniature choices (particularly those carried over from tray to tray), statements, resolution of stories, use of particular characters, and ways these characters change from week to week. I also record the variety of ways that children utilize sand work. For example, some children make a scenario that stands complete at the end of the session, while others make dynamic scenarios and announce, "Okay, let's play now!" These children then move their miniatures around and create a story that has a beginning, middle, and end, requesting clinicians to take roles, have dialogues, or take particular actions. Some children tell elaborate stories about the miniatures in their tray and continue these stories over weeks; other children have little to say about their creations. Some children narrate the development of their sand trays, while others remain silent throughout the process. For some young children (as well as adolescents and adults), clinicians will be able to observe immediate changes in affect with sand therapy; other children approach sand work as they do other things and will move from this activity to others in the room without any particular differences in posture, tone, or affect. Some clients will choose to do sand therapy at each session; others will choose it randomly throughout therapy sessions; and yet still others will select sand therapy to signal that they are interested in working on something to do with difficult emotions.

The older I have gotten, the less I say when children or adults are making sand trays, either alone or with family members. My instruction is always the same: "Use as few or as many miniatures as you wish to make a world in the sand." I often add, "There is no right or wrong way to do this. Whatever you do is just fine." Then I sit back and I witness the process for each individual. I find myself constantly enthralled and curious, and I am finally completely comfortable allowing the process to unfold, because over years I've learned that sand therapy takes its own course. It's completely unique to each person, and I trust that it is providing the individual with whatever he or she needs at that particular time. I firmly believe that with practice, clinicians will learn to trust the process and develop a profound respect for it.

When writing assessment reports for referring parties or courts, I may refer to sand work as a source of information. For example, one 10-year-old African American child, Michael, had developed a range of anxious behaviors after being molested by a cousin (nightmares, tics, clearing his throat, pulling his hair). He made a series of sand worlds with similar themes (see Figures 4.2 and 4.3). I reported on the behaviors observed by parents and teachers, and then added the following paragraph describing the child's creation of scenarios in the sand:

> Michael appears to be acutely anxious and preoccupied with his family's safety. Mother reports that Michael initially confided to her that his cousin threatened to kill him and his parents if Michael told anyone about the abuse. In his play, Michael consistently reveals themes of vulnerability, danger, and fear. For example, when he creates scenarios in the sand, he builds a village he describes as "happy and safe," and he includes houses, playgrounds, trees, farm animals grazing, etc. However, he takes great care to bury snakes, lizards, "poisonous" spiders, and "scuba-diving men with explosives on their backs." He then states that these objects are "always lurking around," and that "they are quiet as mice," but "the family can't protect against them because they don't know they are there." In recent weeks, the number of buried objects has decreased, and

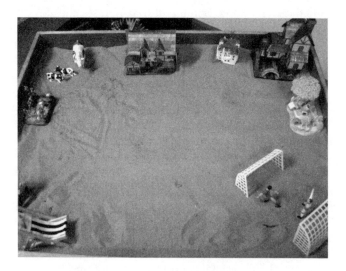

FIGURE 4.2. Michael's anxious worlds.

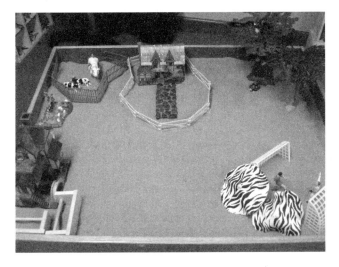

FIGURE 4.3. Michael's resources.

Michael has added safety measures such as fences and walls around the house; these appear to be keeping the danger at a greater distance than before. This change in his sand scenarios appears consistent with parental reports that Michael is sleeping better and has started going outside to play with his friends. Michael is struggling with restoring a sense of safety and security.

Both historical and contemporary uses of sand therapy have been well documented (Turner, 2005; Mitchell & Friedman, 1994), and efforts have been undertaken to create a standardized sand play assessment process (Mielcke, 2005; Sjolund & Schaefer, 1994).

Color Your Feelings

Several techniques that involve using colors as a way of understanding children's emotional states have been documented. For example, O'Connor (1983) describes the Color Your Life technique, and Crisci, Lay, and Lowenstein (1997) use a barometer that children fill with colors.

The Color Your Feelings technique (Hopkins, Huici, & Bermudez, 2005) also draws upon children's ability to show emotional states by using color; however, it requires children first to make very clear associations between colors and emotions, and later to use their specific color–emotion palette to indicate visually their feelings about important relationships (Figure 4.4). I utilize this technique by first asking a child to "list the feelings you have most of the time." These feelings are placed on the right-

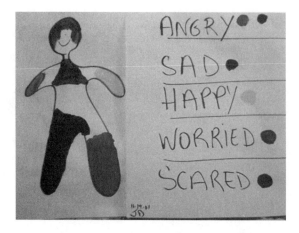

FIGURE 4.4. A color–emotion palette.

hand side of a sheet of easel paper. I then place a small box next to each word and ask the child to "choose the color that best shows that feeling." The child fills in the boxes with the colors he or she chooses (Figure 4.5).

After a child has thus created a color–emotion palette, I make a gingerbread figure to represent a particular person in the child's life. I then ask the child to use the colors to show what feelings, and how much of the feelings, he or she has about this person. I may also make two ginger bread figures to represent two people, and ask the child to show me his or her feelings about being with one person or the other. In Figure 4.6, for

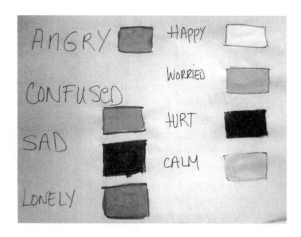

FIGURE 4.5. A Color Your Feelings chart.

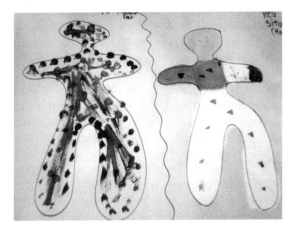

FIGURE 4.6. June's colors/feelings about alleged offender and caretaker.

example, June, an 8-year old Hispanic girl, used her color palette to show how she felt when she was with her mother and how she felt when she was with her alleged offender (her grandfather). The child's art showed a clear contrast, which she had trouble verbalizing because of her feelings of loyalty toward her grandfather. Even in this black-and-white reproduction, you can see the difference between the types and amounts of colors shown, as well as the way in which those colors are used.

This art activity presents the clinician with an interesting way to "see" how a child perceives his or her feelings in the context of relationships with important caretakers. As with any other art therapy technique, this one can be used both as an assessment method and as a bridge to therapeutic dialogue. Very young children as well as older adolescents can accomplish this task.

Other Art Therapy Tools

Among my greatest concerns in working with sexual abuse is the misapplication of art-based information during evaluations. As a consultant to many professionals over the last three decades, I have been concerned with the number of professionals who take liberties with very limited information about art therapy. For example, I frequently hear professionals base conclusions that child sexual abuse occurred on the presence of multiple windows or chimneys, or on the inclusion of "a trauma hole" in a child's tree. We must be very careful not to use a child's art alone to rule in or rule out sexual abuse, although the presence of consistent or obvious art features may suggest a need for further evaluation of possible abuse.

We need to take a conservative view when using children's art; in particular, we must not under- or overrespond to images created during single sessions, or rely too heavily on external interpretation. Projective techniques in particular have not been shown to detect child sexual abuse (Garb, Wood, & Nezworski, 2000; Palmer et al., 2000), and the confirmation of child sexual abuse through sole reliance on children's drawings is not possible (Cohen-Liebman, 1999). Art therapy procedures can yield valuable information however, and can be part of the data-gathering process as well as the treatment process.

There are a number of formal art therapy tools (Oster & Gould Crone, 2004) that attempt to evaluate drawings from a variety of domains. These formal tools have been designed and researched by art therapists and continue to be refined. They are taught to art therapists in art therapy programs across the country, and some are best utilized with formal training. In the field of psychology, most clinicians are familiar with a variety of standard art therapy tools, such as the House–Tree–Person and the Draw-A-Person. However, these projective tests have received negative evidence of their usefulness in favor of more global rating scales (Kaplan, 2003).

Self-Portrait

As just mentioned, the Draw-A-Person has been viewed as limited because it is a projective tool. I find it a little more helpful to be more directive with children and ask them to "draw a picture of yourself." When I ask for a self-portrait, the child is likely to become somewhat introspective and make a picture that is associated with his or her self-image at that particular moment in time. I have found it most useful to get at least three self-portraits during my work with children, because their self-image can be grossly distorted by daily life events (academic performance, altercations with peers, being chosen to participate in a project or ignored, etc.). Once a self-portrait is generated, a clinician can glean a subjective view of its emotional content, evaluate the developmental aspects of the drawing, ask the child to say a little about the picture, and note any features of the drawing that may be unusual. Obviously, the more formal training clinicians have in art therapy, the greater the utility of any type of art for assessment or treatment purposes.

Peterson and Hardin (1997) have developed a screening inventory that allows clinicians to look at children's drawings (self-portraits) and endorse the presence of certain variables, such as encapsulation (when children put a square or circle around the figure) or concealment of genitalia. I have used this screening tool before and after group therapy sessions, to study changes in children's self-portraits. The screening instrument enables a numerical value to be given to each picture, and we hope to see the number decrease as children feel better about themselves or their situation. Again, I emphasize that this instrument (for any other art therapy tool) cannot be used to rule in or rule out child sexual abuse. However, it can help clinicians organize their thoughts and perceptions as they look at children's art. This is an adjunctive or ancillary strategy that is best used within the context of comprehensive assessment and treatment.

Kinetic Family Drawing

Kinetic Family Drawing is a well-documented art therapy tool that is used by individual and family therapists alike as an indicator of a child's view of family relationships (Burns & Kaufman, 1972). This type of drawing usually gives clinicians insights into children's perceptions of closeness and distance, absences, preferred activities, and other related issues (e.g., increased interest in one vs. another family member, or dislikes or likes of specific persons). In common with the other techniques mentioned above, the Kinetic Family Drawing allows the clinician to express therapeutic curiosity about the child's thoughts and feelings. Other art therapy tools that I utilize routinely, and that I believe have the potential to provide substantial information, include Person Picking an Apple from a Tree (Gantt & Tabone, 2003) and Draw a Person in the Rain (Oster & Gould, 1987).

Symbol Work

Often children seem reluctant to do "talk therapy," or they simply are so young that they are not comfortable doing so. Other children (or older people) are so prone to overuse language that it is difficult to gauge their emotional states or prioritize what's important to them. In any or all of these instances, it is useful to "cut to the chase" with a very simple exercise that most people will thoroughly enjoy.

For instance, I was working with Caroline, a Hispanic 13-year-old who was having a bad day. She came into my office, plopped herself in the chair, and announced, "I'm not into talking today. I had a rotten day, and I'm tired." I empathized by noting that "everyone has days like this." She looked away and seemed mostly angry. "No worries," I said. "I won't ask you to talk when you don't feel like it." I got up, moved over to the play therapy room, and motioned for her to follow. "I've got an idea. Look around the shelves, or anywhere in the room. I'd like you to find a miniature that best shows the 'rotten day' that you just had, and then find a couple of things that might help you deal with the rotten day." It took her about 10 minutes to find two miniatures that represented her rotten day. These were two dolls, a boy and a girl, whom she placed in close proximity to each other; she also placed a group of brown-skinned children in one group and a group of white, blond children in another group, with a wall between them (see Figure 4.7).

This led to a discussion about her crush on this particular boy and her worries that she was "not his type" (she was dark-skinned and dark-haired). She worried that the boy she liked only liked blond, blue-eyed girls. We spent some time talking about cultural identity and her comfort with her brown skin and eyes. I introduced the idea that there were lots of different "looks" and that she would be pleasing to some boys and not to others, just as she would like and not like boys for similar or different reasons. I decided to read her a book about racial differences later on, and we then moved to talking about how she might continue to feel better.

When I asked her to pick a miniature that showed something that would help her with her rotten day, she picked a table, chairs, and some fruit, setting up a little dinner table (Figure 4.8). She noted that she was going out to dinner with her father tonight, and that she would have fun going out with him: "He always makes me feel really special, like we're going out on a real date." This child had spent the session talking about her rotten day, and had refocused and looked forward to an experience that would cause her to feel happy. She had identified some of her self-

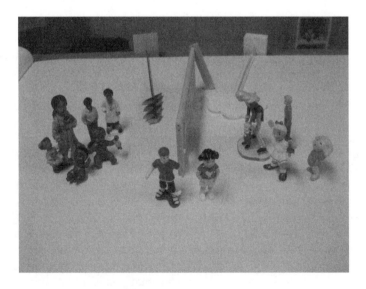

FIGURE 4.7. Caroline's bad day.

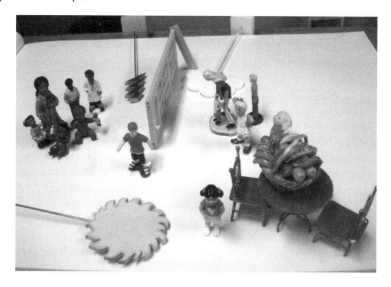

FIGURE 4.8. Help with Caroline's bad day.

image concerns at school and her current worries about boys liking her, and we had talked about how to cope with difficult experiences/ emotions. We'd then shifted to talking about how to feel better (less rejected), and she was able to identify her supportive relationship with her father as a resource for herself.

I have used symbol work with groups and families in very specific ways. For example, when the sniper crisis of 2002 occurred in the Washington, D.C., metropolitan area, the anxiety level was understandably very high in all my coworkers. A number of meetings were held to discuss how our personal anxiety was affecting our work relationships and our clients. These were very helpful meetings, except that some people did not feel as comfortable as others did about speaking in groups. Instead, I offered times for people to come to my office and work with symbols. I asked group members first to find miniatures that showed their thoughts and feelings about the crisis that was going on, and then to place those miniatures in a smaller circle inside a larger circle.

After they placed all the symbols of crisis inside the inner circle, I asked them to "find a miniature that best shows the first and second and third step in responding to this crisis—in other words, some possible help or support that might occur in response to the crisis." The final result depicted the crisis as contained or surrounded by symbols of hope, healing, recovery, and resiliency. Those who attended these meetings found this exercise helpful, and a few commented that these images seemed to "stay with them" for quite a long time. One woman commented that she had a dream that included some of the miniatures.

Combining Verbal Communication with Expressive Strategies

Some children are very adept at verbal communication and seem to enjoy sitting with their therapists, talking, sharing information, and responding to questions. Even when this type of open and facile verbal communication occurs, I still encourage experimenting with expressive arts from time to time, just to amplify, complement, or augment what is being said. These youth tend to enjoy expressive work and often are capable of great insight about their creations. In addition, some highly verbal youth need to develop a comfort level with expressive strategies. The degree of receptivity or noncompliance they exhibit to such strategies can itself be informative.

Play, Puppet, Storytelling, and Dramatic Play

Play therapy offices are usually equipped with puppets and with games and toys for storytelling and dramatic play. All of these techniques can be useful to children and may be employed more or less often, depending on their age and personality (Gerity, 1999; Weber & Haen, 2005). Puppets, for example, can be used by both boys and girls, and in individual, group, or family therapy environments. Puppets can facilitate communication, can spark creative storytelling, or can become instant invitations to create and act out plays. Clinicians must remain tuned in to thematic material, repetition of themes, and the ways stories evolve and get resolved. Chapter Nine discusses a young client whose puppet play served as the pivotal strategy for revealing and processing her feelings about maternal abandonment.

The use of these three techniques cannot be overemphasized as an opportunity for children to take active roles in shaping stories that may symbolically reveal inner concerns and distress. By creating stories and acting them out, children can literally change their perceptions of personal mastery and control. This occurs through their physical movement, attention to detail, narration of a story that might reflect internal concerns, and ability to alter the outcome of such a story (by a change from passive to active mode). These three forms of play therapy are most helpful to children who can use fantasy to compensate for real losses and for those who can discover new options and possibilities, creating a sense of hope.

INTEGRATING EXPRESSIVE THERAPIES AND FAMILY WORK

Play therapy, and other expressive therapies as well, can be incorporated with family therapy sessions (Riley & Malchiodi, 2003; Combs & Freedman, 1990). In my experience, however, many family therapists seem skeptical, hesitant, or ambivalent about using such therapies in their work with families with young children. In fact, some family therapists have questioned the apparent exclusion of young children from family therapy. Green (1994) finds three reasons that might explain this exclusion: some family therapists' inability to relate to children as individuals; the fact that the most influential leaders in the family therapy field were most interested in adults and suggested indirect treatment of children; and some family therapists' lack of basic training and confidence in how to work with children, even when they are motivated to do so. This exclusion continues to be the status quo, despite active and visible encouragement from respected leaders such as Carl Whitaker and Virginia Satir, and recent efforts to promote a crossover between the fields of play therapy and family therapy (Schaefer & Carey, 1994; Gil, 1994). Sadly, neither play (and other expressive) therapists nor family therapists routinely exchange or promote their ideas, strategies, and approaches—partly due to some unwillingness among members of both groups to receive yet more training, and/or because the techniques of one group are viewed by the other with skepticism (as undesirable or impractical).

ESTABLISHMENT OF PROFESSIONAL
STANDARDS FOR EXPRESSIVE THERAPIES

By now, groups of clinicians who provide art, play, and sand therapies have instituted professional standards by creating associations and governing and credentialing boards, developing respected journals, and sponsoring annual conferences. Membership in these professional associations has grown over the last two decades, as have high-quality training programs, scientific research, and increased status.

ART THERAPY

The American Art Therapy Association (AATA) was founded in 1969 and has approximately 4,750 members. In 1970, the AATA began to provide certification for registered art therapists, and the certification function is now provided by the Art Therapy Credential Board (founded in 1993). There are currently approximately 3,000 registered art therapists.

Play Therapy

The Association for Play Therapy (APT) was founded in 1982 and currently has over 5,400 members. Guidelines for becoming a registered play therapist were developed in 1994, and currently there are approximately 620 registered play therapists and 340 registered play therapist supervisors.

Sand Therapy

The International Society for Sandplay Therapy (ISST) was founded by Dora Kalff in 1985, with the help of several international colleagues. Membership in the ISST currently numbers approximately 60 members worldwide, is open to qualified therapists, and is based on a certification process. In the United States, Weinrib and Bradway have been strong leaders in the development of Sandplay Therapists of America, which publishes a journal twice yearly called the *Journal of Sandplay Therapy* (Mitchell & Friedman, 1994).

SUMMARY

Those working with children, particularly child victims of sexual abuse or other forms of maltreatment, recognize their natural reluctance to speak about what's happened to them, how they feel, how they think about things, and how they feel the injuries affect them. Young children in particular have greater difficulty with perceiving such events accurately and reporting them in ways that are clear in meaning. Children have a much broader way of communicating that doesn't rely on their verbal repertoires, and thus clinicians seeking to understand children need to become conversant in expressive strategies.

"Expressive therapies" is a term that includes the therapeutic use of many different expressive techniques, such as visual/manual arts and crafts, play, sand therapy, drama, dance/movement, writing, music, and many more. Pioneering professionals have sought to create a bridge between the expressive arts and mental health; they recognize and honor the many curative and abreactive powers of expressive communication.

In this chapter, special emphasis has been placed on art, play, and sand therapies, since children tend to have a particular affinity for these therapies. However, many other creative interventions are possible. Indeed, many professionals who work with children and adolescents find it necessary to develop a broad repertoire of engaging, dynamic, and creative activities in order to elicit children's attention and participation. The expressive therapies have much to contribute and can be easily integrated with other, more traditional strategies. Case studies further illustrate the potential uses of expressive therapies in work with traumatized children (Gil, 2003b); four such case studies are included in the second part of this book. Finally, readers are encouraged to read the ample literature on expressive therapies and obtain additional training in them, in order to maximize their potential to be useful to children and their families.

5

Cognitive-Behavioral Therapy

In the current mental health care environment, there is great pressure to utilize empirically based therapies. A recent text (Christophersen & Mortweet, 2001) evaluates and summarizes "treatments that work" with children. More and more often, funding sources, insurance companies, parents, and mental health professionals themselves look for methodologies whose success has been substantiated by research. Several aspects of this situation are noteworthy: (1) Most mental health professionals in private practice or agency settings do not have the time or the resources to conduct research regarding treatment outcome; (2) the validation of certain approaches through research does not automatically discount those methods that have not had the benefit of empirical study; and (3) the knowledge base of the present book's topic (treatment of abused/traumatized children in general and sexually abused children in particular) is still evolving. Nevertheless, mental health practitioners must commit themselves resolutely to creating climates in which research is integrated into their practices. This will advance everyone's understanding of the potential benefits of therapy, and will respond to scholarly pleas for additional research that supports and guides the effectiveness of mental health services.

Probably the most well-researched approaches have been behavioral and cognitive-behavioral strategies. Reinecke, Dattilio, and Freeman (1996) note:

> Cognitive therapy with children, as in work with adults, is founded upon the assumption that behavior is adaptive, and that there is an interaction

between an individual's thoughts, feelings, and behaviors. The major thrust of cognitive-behavioral therapy is toward understanding the nature and development of an individual's behavior repertoire and the accompanying cognitive processes. (p. 2)

The earliest and most famous behavioral study was conducted on dogs by the Russian psychologist Ivan Pavlov the early years of the 20th century. Pavlov demonstrated that learning could occur through "classical conditioning" (i.e., associating an initially unrelated stimulus with a behavior by pairing that stimulus with another one that did elicit the behavior). He and later behaviorists believed that desired behaviors could be shaped through reinforcement, and that negative behaviors could be extinguished through some type of manipulation of consequences. These studies were more effective in that specific variables were visibly manipulated, provided, or withheld. Eventually, the principles of learning theory promoted by behaviorists were applied to a number of specific problems (e.g., phobias), and treatment outcome studies showed effectiveness.

The behavioral therapies were later adjusted to include dimensions of cognition and affect, so that the term "cognitive-behavioral therapy" (CBT) is more frequently utilized today. The additional focus of cognitive therapy encourages clinicians to identify and address cognitive distortions or thinking errors, thoughts that are illogical or bizarre but which unduly influence negative behaviors. These problematic thoughts occur frequently in abused children who may believe, for example, that the abuse is their fault because they didn't say no or fight off their abuser.[1] Children are vulnerable to developing thinking errors due to limited cognitive skills and perceptions (given developmental immaturity) as well as their desire to protect their idealized images of parents whom they love and trust. In the face of a parent who reassures a child that sexual abuse is secret and a loving expression between parent and child, children can be vulnerable to developing alternate explanations in which they take full responsibility for the abuse.

Ellis (1962) and Beck (1976) are often given credit for conceptualizing the need for cognitive restructuring in which negative or distorted think-

---

[1] In our rush to reassure children that the abuse is not their fault, we sometimes overlook a careful exploration of the child's understanding of why s/he is to blame. I therefore encourage a slow and careful review of "what the child says to him/herself about what happened," or "how the child would explain what happened to someone else." Once the reasoning is clear, therapists can attempt to provide alternative information in order to challenge the child's misconception.

ing patterns are challenged and revised. The term CBT signals an expanded interest in the interactions among affect (what individuals feel), cognitions (what thoughts they associate with feelings), and behaviors (how those feelings and subsequent thoughts affect what actions are taken and vice-versa), as well as the contextual piece (socioenvironmental issues). Although the application of CBT seems similar for children and adults, working with children requires therapists to "carefully attend to the interpersonal contexts in which children's beliefs and attitudes are acquired, as well as the developmental factors associated with behavioral and emotional change" (Reinecke, Dattilio, & Freeman, 1996, p. 9). In cases of familial child sexual abuse, there are obvious reasons to work with children's families to challenge the child's attributions about the abuse. Cohen and Mannarino (2002) discuss the relationship between attribution and symptom formation, the role of shame, the complexity of self-blame, external blame, perpetrator blame, and the importance of maximizing therapists' ability to encourage expression of idiosyncratic attributions (e.g., using standardized instruments).

As mentioned earlier in this text, CBT has been found to be effective in the treatment of sexually abused children (Cohen & Mannarino, 1993, 1996, 1997, 1998; Cohen, Mannarino, Berliner, & Deblinger, 2000; Deblinger, McLeer, & Henry, 1990; Deblinger, Stauffer, & Steer, 2001; Deblinger, Steer, & Lippmann, 1999; Saywitz, Mannarino, Berliner, & Cohen, 2000). The research clearly substantiates these strategies as helpful in decreasing the symptoms these children commonly experienced. CBT strategies are also utilized effectively with other populations—for example, impulsive children (Kendall & Braswell, 1993).

Deblinger and Heflin (1996) promote CBT strategies as having multiple rewards specifically for sexually abused children and their families. They articulate a model that appears to be successful in decreasing children's symptoms, particularly those symptoms related to PTSD. The basic elements of Deblinger and Heflin's approach with children include "modeling; coping skills training; gradual exposure; cognitive and affective processing; and education regarding sexual abuse, healthy sexuality, and personal safety skills" (p. 49). They further note that of these, the most important components are gradual exposure and affective processing. Their work with parents has three major components: "social skills training . . . gradual exposure . . . and behavior management skills" (p. 114). Knell (1993) integrates play therapy with CBT strategies in order to make this approach possible with even preschool children, and has also described her use of cognitive-behavioral play therapy specifically with sexually abused children (Knell & Ruma, 1996).

In addition to Deblinger and Heflin's work, Cohen et al. (2000) have made a substantial contribution to understanding the applicability of

CBT approaches to helping sexually abused children and their families. Their structured model of trauma-focused CBT (TF-CBT) has been well studied and duplicated, and, like Deblinger and Heflin's model, it includes parental participation in psychoeducational groups. It also includes individual child therapy, groups for children, and child–parent sessions.

CBT has obvious theoretical and practical strengths, and it has been validated as a treatment of choice for adult victims of trauma (Foa & Rothbaum, 1998). For a child population, however, it has some obvious limitations, because it depends heavily on clients' abilities to utilize cognitive functions, reasoning, awareness, accountability, impulse control, and willingness to alter behaviors. Young children, for example, may not be great candidates for a verbally based program, although they will certainly respond to external conditioning of their problem behaviors. In other words, a desired change in a child's behavior may be achieved, but this may occur in isolation from (or with very limited) understanding or true processing. The child may still be suppressing unprocessed traumatic material that is at risk for resurfacing in the future.

For example, if a child is bedwetting due to emotional upheaval, and behavioral approaches manage to effect a change, it's possible that the original emotional issues may be exhibited in other symptoms (immediately or over the long term), or that the emotional concerns remain vulnerable to resurfacing at a later time through either the original or an alternate symptom. Marnie was a 4-year-old child whose bedwetting appeared during her struggles to cope with sexual abuse by her older sister who was sneaking into her bedroom at night. Her parents took her to a pediatrician who referred her for behavioral therapy, which was quite effective: Marnie stopped urinating in her bed. Unfortunately, her sister continued to come into her room at night for another week until Marnie was referred to me for generic play therapy. The mother was concerned that the family's recent relocation had taken a toll on this child. Marnie kept bringing up a "monster" who woke her up and touched her privates and then hid under her bed. When I asked her to draw a picture of the monster, she drew her older sister, Maggie—who (as we later discovered) was being sexually abused by an aunt.

My point is that although CBT is grounded in good theory and is empirically based, it still may be of limited usefulness in helping some sexually abused children. When discussing future research directions, Cohen et al. (2000) urge attention to the specific TF-CBT components that might be more or less useful when offered separately or in combination with other components, as well as to specific demographic subgroups that respond better (e.g., children of different genders, ethnicities, or ages). In addition, they state that "it is important to identify which children do not respond well to trauma-focused CBT interventions and to empirically evaluate alternative psychosocial, pharmacologic, or combination treatments that may help such children recover from traumatic exposure" (p. 1218).

The purpose of the present text is to promote combination treatments as potentially effective with sexually abused children, and to encourage research that distinguishes the benefits of CBT or TF-CBT from the benefits of cognitive-behavioral play therapy, which appears to be provided routinely in the course of providing these versions of CBT. Deblinger and Heflin (1996), for example, in describing a proper therapy setting, suggest providing a small selection of toys, including paper, crayons, toy telephones, dolls, puppets, and a feelings chart depicting different emotions. The presence of these therapeutic toys indicates that art and play are ingredients of their model of CBT. It's also clear that these toys are used as props to promote therapy goals, and that their use is not considered therapeutic in and of themselves (in contrast to the use of toys by play therapists). Finally, Deblinger and Heflin (1996) caution clinicians to avoid making their therapy offices overstimulating or distracting through an overabundance of toys.

As noted above, the primary components of Deblinger and Heflin's work are gradual exposure and affective processing for children, and social skills training, gradual exposure, and behavior management for their parents. Expressive therapies, as discussed in Chapters Four and Six of the present book, also focus on gradual exposure and affective work. However, these occur in different forms: They are initiated by children or facilitated by clinicians and employed at their pace, within the context of a therapy relationship, and with respect for children's need to utilize their defensive mechanisms in a fluid fashion. It appears that the primary difference between these two types of approaches is that trauma-focused play therapy (TF-PT) allow for natural healing mechanisms to go into effect at a child's own pace. By contrast, CBT or TF-CBT seeks to introduce a set agenda that may or may not be inviting or comfortable for children—particularly those sexually abused children in denial, with fragmented memories, or with suppressed and compartmentalized memories. The new scientific evidence about brain development also indicates that traumatic events are experienced and/or stored in the right hemisphere of the brain; this suggests that allowing children a period of time to access or stimulate the right hemisphere of the brain could eventually activate the necessary functions of the left hemisphere, which appear to shut down during traumatic experiences. Stimulating right hemisphere activity through expressive, nonverbal modalities is thus worthwhile and relevant in our work with traumatized individuals. (See Chapters One and Three). At the same time, expressive therapies may be criticized for prioritizing the therapy relationship, inviting nonverbal processing, and allowing children to (sometimes) maintain denial, which may exacerbate symptoms. Another possible criticism of play therapy or other expressive therapies is the traditional exclusion of parents, which in cases of sexual abuse will be problematic and short-sighted. I believe that any treatment model with sexually abused children must include collaboration with parents though a variety of services, including (but not limited to) coaching, individual therapy for parents if necessary, psychoeducational groups, parent–child therapies, home-based services, crisis intervention services, and family therapy.

Having stated my bias toward integrated work that includes both directive and nondirective strategies, I must also emphasize that some clinical situations warrant CBT interventions without delay. These include physical and sexual aggression in children, work with victims of violent rapes, as well as active suicidal thoughts and plans. In these cases, there may be identifiable target behaviors and the assessment phase can be modified in order to allow for immediate and specific CBT interventions.

CASE ILLUSTRATION: CURTIS

Curtis, an 11-year-old European American child, was referred to therapy after his parents walked in on him while he was sexually abusing his 4-year-old sister. Given his age, his excuse that his sister "forced him" to have sex with her seemed more than implausible. Curtis's parents opted to contact child protective services (CPS), but because Curtis had not been in a caretaker role with his sister, the parents were encouraged to call the police. A detective interviewed Mr. and Mrs. Anderson about what they had seen, and then spoke directly to Curtis, who persisted in denying any wrongdoing. He continued to insist not only that his sister had initiated contact with him, but that she had eventually put his penis in her mouth. Of course, the detective kept Curtis talking until he eventually revealed that he had tried to penetrate her anus with his fingers—something Mrs. Anderson thought that she had seen. Detective Scott told Mr. and Mrs. Anderson that they had to get Curtis into therapy immediately, and also noted that he would be continuing his investigation. The Andersons talked it over and called me the very next day.

Intake Session

Mr. and Mrs. Anderson seemed appropriately concerned, teary, and distressed about their daughter, Norma. They wanted help for both their children, and they emphasized that Curtis was as much a priority as

Norma. In spite of the fact that they recognized that Norma had been victimized by her much larger and older brother, they were also worried about what would make Curtis "do such a hidious thing."

I took a psychosocial history of the family. Mr. and Mrs. Anderson depicted themselves as involved parents who held themselves partially responsible for Curtis's problems. They went on to elaborate on that statement by sharing that they had felt suspicious of Curtis since he was very small, and that they treated him differently from their daughter. Upon further examination it became apparent that there was a family secret of some sort, and I continued my interview with an uncomfortable awareness that I was asking questions with unusual caution and discomfort. Both parents worked outside the home.

The Andersons continued to describe themselves as good parents who had learned a lot by the mistakes they had made with Curtis. They said that there were a lot of stressful things going on when Curtis was a small child, and that they were nervous and irritable with him. They described Curtis as "fussy" and "demanding." The father added, "Not much has changed since then." They talked about a difficult pregnancy and delivery, and their perception of their children as "night and day." In fact, both of them changed their facial expressions and tone of voice when they spoke of one or the other child. Norma was described in positive terms, and their faces lit up when they talked about the joy she had brought to their lives. Conversely, talk of Curtis was imbedded with tension, passive–aggressive humor, and discernible disdain. Slowly but surely, they described the context in which the sexual abuse had occurred.

As I talked with the Anderson couple about their children's development, their different attitudes toward the two youngsters persisted in their descriptions. Curtis, they stated, had many social and behavioral problems, while Norma got along with everyone, was well behaved, and excelled at anything she tried to do—particularly painting and riding her bicycle. As a matter of fact, they used bicycle riding as a way to emphasize their difficulties with Curtis. "Curtis wanted us to come outside every moment of the day and night to watch him ride his bike. He was almost vicious in the way he insisted that we come out, no matter what we were doing. Eventually, he became so loud and disruptive that we had to go out and watch him ride his bike." Mrs. Anderson added that she thought that Curtis pretended to fall just to get a little sympathy. They quickly added, "Norma learned to ride the bike quickly, and then she rode around the back patio by herself, being careful not to crash into anything. She always listened to us so well . . . When Curt wasn't trying to get us to come out and stare at him riding his bike, he would disappear somewhere, even though we repeated over and over that he had to stay in the yard." Mr. Anderson underscored his wife's statement by noting that Curt would sometimes fall down just to get attention, and that he would often yell so that the neighbors would eventually look out their window.

"Maybe if he had had friends," Mrs. Anderson noted, "things would have been easier . . . he just seemed underfoot all the time, and we couldn't find anyone that he would get along with."

Curtis was currently attending a public elementary school, and he was in the fourth grade. His mother commented, "I guess you're not surprised to hear he was held back a grade." I asked the parents if they knew why the school had held him back, and they said, "They told us he just wasn't maturing at the same pace as other children. His grades were marginal, and they could have passed him to the next grade, but they decided it would be better for him to repeat the grade."

When I asked how they viewed this decision currently, they said that Curtis had gotten worse after being held back, because he felt that other kids made fun of him and that he was smarter and bigger than most of his classmates. "He thinks he's better-looking too, which is a joke." I found Mr. Anderson's comment odd, and I pursued this a little bit. "Tell me what you think about his physical appearance." "Well," he responded, "he's certainly not the best-looking person in the family." I anticipated that Norma would be described differently; sure enough, both parents gushed as they talked about her bright eyes, the way people stopped them on the street to comment on how stunning she was, and their perception that "everyone fell in love with her immediately." I began to realize that Curtis was probably able to discern his parents' feelings toward him as clearly as I did in this initial session.

When I inquired about the sexual abuse of Norma, their eyes teared up immediately, and they seemed angry and distressed at what Curtis had done to Norma. "We really want to know what's wrong with him," the mother supplicated, "and I want to make very sure that my daughter is going to be safe." I asserted that Norma's safety was critical, as was trying to understand what was going on with Curtis. I recommended individual therapy for both children, followed by conjoint sibling sessions once their individual therapists felt that these would be appropriate. I also told Mr. and Mrs. Anderson that they would be expected to attend a group for parents of sexually aggressive children, as well as to participate in family therapy as required by the children's therapists. "In addition," I stated firmly, "it's critical that you follow all our recommendations about monitoring Curtis, making sure the children are not left unsupervised at any time, and taking other measures to make sure that Norma will not be abused again." I reviewed some guidelines that they needed to implement immediately, and I gave them a written reminder. Finally, I told them to tell both children that they were coming to see a counselor who works with children who have had "touching problems" (i.e., touching of the private parts).

Initial Sessions with Curtis

Curtis was a sullen, unfriendly, awkward child who seemed surly by design. I had the feeling that he was acting a role and didn't really know how he felt about coming to see a therapist. He would alternately act cool, rude, and somewhat vulnerable and sweet. He told me as he walked in, "I've done this before, so don't be asking me a lot of questions." "You've done what before?" I asked. He said, "Stupid therapy . . . I used to go to a weirdo guy who kept staring at me and asked lots of questions." "Oh," I said, "you've had experience seeing a therapist." "Yeah," he said in a louder tone, "and you aren't tricking me into talking."

"Sure," I said, "you can say as much or as little as you'd like." Then I showed him around my room and waited to see what he was interested in doing. "By the way," I asked, "what did your mom and dad tell you about coming to see me?" "Nothin'!" he stated firmly. "Oh, OK, well then let me tell you a little about coming to see me." He looked away. "Your mom told me that she walked into your bedroom and found you touching Norma's private parts." "I did *not* do that!" he shouted. "Well, that's what your mom told me she saw, and what you're saying is that you didn't touch her. That happens a lot, you know." "What?" he asked. I looked at him and said, "Kids who touch other kids in their private parts don't like people to know they did that." Curtis stopped and seemed curious about what I'd said. "Do you see other kids—I mean kids who do that?" "Yes," I said, "lots of kids who touch other kids' private parts . . . so many kids that we're writing a book just for kids who touch private parts." "That's gross," he said. "Is it going to have pictures?" I wasn't sure if he was making an inappropriate joke or if he was challenging me. I kept my composure and stated, "What do you think . . . would pictures be a good idea?" "Forget it," he said, and we moved on to his active exploration of the room.

By the end of this first session, Curtis had looked at the miniatures (especially the soldiers), and he had asked a lot of questions: who bought all my toys, whether he could take things home, and whether his sister was going to come to this room too. He looked up when I told him that his sister would be seeing a different counselor. "How many times do I have to come here?" he asked on his way out. "Good question," I responded as he walked down the stairs in front of me.

At the following session, I told Curtis that we were going to divide the time into two parts, and he could decide what part he wanted to do first. "We need to work on the touching problem for half of the session," I stated as he rolled his eyes, "and the other half you will be able to play with whatever you like in here . . . Which one do you want to do first?" He responded very quickly and definitely: "I wanna play first!" We set a time period (30 minutes) for play, after which I would stop him so that we could do some work on the touching problem. I would tackle this problem in directive fashion, because his behavior needed to be brought under control as soon as possible. My understanding of the problem was that Curtis's internal controls weren't working, and that he needed external controls until we could figure out how to engage the part of himself that could control problem behaviors at will.

Predictably, Curtis didn't want to stop playing, but I had set a timer, so there was little room for discussion. "When the bell rings," I stated," it is time to stop and work on the touching problem." I had selected a videotape for him to watch in an attempt to begin teasing out his thinking about his inappropriate behaviors. I find that providing education as a way to engage children in dialogue—or, at the very least, cognitive reevaluation of established ideas—is likely to be more effective than asking children (especially boys) about their feelings. In my experience, boys tend to develop compensatory anger as a way to avoid their underlying feelings of helplessness; thus they require treatment that addresses their aggressive behaviors and encourages feelings of empowerment (Crenshaw & Mordock, 2005).

Once the timer bell rang, I told Curtis that we'd be watching a videotape entitled *Three Kinds of Touches* (Pennsylvania Coalition against Rape, n.d.). This tape reviews three kinds of touches: safe touches, "ouch" touches, and "uh-oh" touches. In other words, it reviews loving, safe, and nurturing touches; hurtful touches, including aggression or violence; and touching of the private parts that can make children feel uncomfortable or confused. Curtis was able to repeat the lesson types and describe situations he had encountered that would demonstrate each type of touching. He didn't elaborate much in his answers and managed to convey his indifference to these lessons, but he also cooperated and volunteered some (minimal) information. He asked whether we would have to see that "stupid tape" again, and I told him that once was usually enough for most kids. I told him we'd do some other activities in our next session, and he said emphatically, "You mean after I get my free time."

Subsequent Sessions

The following four sessions were focused on developing a comfort level with verbalization of sexual issues, as well as establishing the basic lessons that would be repeated throughout the course of therapy. We reviewed the ThinkTool Kit cards (Smith & Nelson, n.d.), a set of cards that

I've used successfully when tackling the problem behavior of sexual aggression in children. I first reviewed the 30 or so cards with Curtis, simply asking him what he thought each picture meant and how it might pertain to the problem behavior in question. After reviewing the cards and in some cases clarifying their meaning, I asked him to choose a few that he found relevant or interesting in any way. I then photocopied each card he had chosen, creating a series of sheets that we then personalized by adding Curtis-specific statements. For example, when we looked at a card that had a STOP sign, we began to talk about what kinds of thoughts or feelings would cue Curtis that he needed to stop and do something (take some kind of action). Curtis was able to describe that when he felt jealous (of his sister) because his parents were paying more attention to her, he began to feel angry, and he noticed that he began "chewing his teeth." I commended Curtis for coming up with a feeling that led to an action. We then role-played as I asked him to pretend to be angry, pretend to "chew his teeth," and then stop and do something else. When we role-played, he was stymied about what to do. Talking with his parents was not an option for him (and my work with the parents did not change this). Instead, he decided that he could go read a book, write in his journal, or draw a cartoon. I modeled stopping and attempting these alternative behaviors; we role-played a typical situation when he might feel angry; and then he practiced new behaviors while I watched and reinforced them. All those options served to relax Curtis and provided him with enough self-comfort that he did not escalate his negative feelings and did not end up acting out in an aggressive way.

Curtis's participation seemed to increase gradually, although he seemed compelled either to miss an appointment from time to time or otherwise communicate his discomfort or lack of interest. At the same time, I also watched Curtis develop an introspection that he lacked when I first met him, as well as a willingness to expose his vulnerabilities.

I read a book with him called *Woody and Willy* (Cabe, 2002). At first, Curtis loudly objected to reading a book for "little kids." When he continued to object, I told him that maybe what we should do together was to use *Woody and Willy* as a point of reference, but instead to translate this material so that older kids would find it more appealing. Curtis was pretty creative and playful during this project, and we both discovered that he was a born teacher. As a matter of fact, he spontaneously fashioned a pointer and pretended to be teaching lessons to kids his age. His tone of voice, expressions, affect, and movement became more expansive as he delved into this task.

I then introduced another book, *STOP: Just for Kids* (Allred & Burns, 1997), and Curtis was pretty impressed to hear that kids with touching problems had written it. We took turns reading pages, and he offered his agreement or disagreement on each chapter. The lessons were starting to kick in, as he was able to repeat them with greater ease. We were still working somewhat on the surface, however, and I knew that this would probably continue until we approached discussion of his own sexual abuse—that is, how he had learned about sex in the first place. This disclosure did not come easily for Curtis; in fact, it was rather accidental. We were playing a card game called Let's Talk about Touching (Johnson, 1992) that has Problem cards (each describing a problem situation) and Solution cards (each suggesting possible solutions for children). Curtis selected a card that said,

> Justin thinks he is bad because his body feels good when Jed, an adult, touches his private parts. He has heard that the older person is wrong. But if the touching feels good, Justin thinks he must be a bad person. What do you think?

When Curtis read this card, it made him blush. I made a mental note that the card described a situation involving an adult male. "What do you think should happen, Curtis?" I asked. "If he tells anybody, that guy might off him!" "What do you mean, 'off him'?" I inquired, and he looked at me and said, "Let's get another card *about somebody else.*" I told Curtis that I was willing to move on at this moment, but I had noticed that something about the card and the situation that was described was difficult for him.

In the next session, Curtis didn't want to play with the cards. I reassured him again that we wouldn't spend a lot of time with the cards, but added that I wanted to say something to him. I weighed my words carefully: "Curtis, there are lots of kids who touch other kids, and most of the time they've learned about this kind of touching and gotten interested in sex because of someone else—someone who taught them about this kind of touching." Curtis would not make eye contact with me at this point. I further noted that "lots of kids, boys especially, feel really embarrassed when these things happen—especially if they've sort of liked what happened or if they feel that they can't tell anyone." Curtis glanced up at me with tears in his eyes, looking very vulnerable and scared: "That happened to me." "What happened to you?" I asked, and he went on to tell me about a neighbor who had sexually abused him. This neighbor had moved away about 2 years ago, but Curtis said he was still scared because this neighbor had told him he would always be watching him from afar.

Over the next 4 months, we would talk about this neighbor "in code," and Curtis maintained a safe distance by always talking about how other kids might think or feel. Curtis asked and explored many questions related to the abuse: Why him? Was he now homosexual? Would other kids be able to tell that he was abused? Would the neighbor go to jail? Why had the neighbor picked him and not some other kid? The most worrisome question was whether he would become "like" his abuser; this question was troubling to navigate because Curtis had, in fact, abused his sister. However, Curtis responded well to information about offending behaviors. He particularly embraced the ideas that he was accountable for his own behavior, and that he could make choices about what to do and not to do. I'll always remember Curtis's face when he would enter the office announcing gleefully that he had thought about doing something inappropriate at school and chose to forgo that in favor of something else. He clearly experienced mastery and personal power as he put some of the therapy lessons to work in real-life situations.

Termination

Curtis participated in therapy for approximately 10 months. During that time, he became accountable for his inappropriate and hurtful behavior to his sister; he wrote and read an apology to his sister, clearly stating that he had been wrong; and he disclosed and addressed his own victimization by an adult male. Curtis responded really well to several CBT strategies, and he and I developed a very comfortable talking relationship. Curtis grew in self-esteem and also seemed to view his parents more realistically—looking less to them for validation, and instead developing lots of internal talking, assertiveness, and self-encouragement.

Predictably, Curtis's parents had very little reaction to his disclosure of sexual abuse. I had learned to anticipate their negative or neutral responses to this child, and I had many theories about what might be eliciting these unusual parental responses. I had hypothesized from the very first (intake) session that there was a disturbance in the parent–child relationships, and each of my interactions with them reinforced this belief further. Although Curtis's parents believed Curtis, they quickly minimized the situation: "Couldn't have been too much of a problem for you, Curt. I remember how much you liked him and how you begged to go over to his house." I had a coaching session with the parents that had minimal impact. They were relentlessly callous toward Curtis, and I noted how defensive he became in their presence. I began to see him as a child in desperate need of positive attention—a child who seemed to respond well to positive individual encouragement from others. His teacher, for example, noted that Curtis had difficult social interactions with peers and seemed to elicit negative attention through his disruptive, in-your-face behaviors. In spite of that, the teacher noted that Curtis had a way about him that kept him likable.

The neighbor's abuse was reported, and when the police investigated, they found that another child in the neighborhood had made allegations of sexual abuse by the same adult. Apparently this allegation and the initiation of a police report were what had precipitated the neighbor's move. Although Mr. and Mrs. Anderson were cooperative with the police, the investigating detective made note of the parents' chastising of Curtis and inquiry about Curtis's potential to become an adult pedophile. Detective Scott had told the parents that treatment was the most important preventive measure for Curtis, and the parents had made a disheartening comment about Curtis's therapy: "I'd feel better if he didn't like going there so much," the mother had quipped.

When I think back on this case, I'm very grateful for the opportunity both to work with Curtis and to reflect on the improvements he made in his own self-understanding, self-control, and self-image. At the same time, I regret my inability to make more headway with Mr. and Mrs. Anderson, who refused to attend group therapy, canceled most appointments with me, and continued to view their child in a skeptical way. The parents never revealed whatever secret they were harboring, and this case—more than almost any other clinical situation—left me feeling uneasy and concerned, because I was unable to find a way to improve this child's relationship with his parents. I remain satisfied, however, with Curtis's use of his therapy experience to gain insight about the effects of his feelings on his thoughts about himself and his behavior toward others. The fact that we have not heard from this family again also gives me optimism about Curtis's ability to control his aggressive sexual impulses with his sibling.

CASE ILLUSTRATION: ESPERANZA

Esperanza was a 6-year-old Hispanic child who had been sexually abused by her stepfather. She came from a family with few financial resources. Her mother, Elena, worked in a cafeteria for part of the day and cleaned a building at night. Elena's husband, Raul, worked at construction sites whenever he could and maintained a serious drinking habit, usually depleting Elena's income quickly. Because Elena was the primary breadwinner, Raul spent much time at home—ostensibly taking care of Elena's two small children, Esperanza and 5-year-old Claudio (both from a previous common-law relationship with a man named Alvaro).

Elena's own history was horrific. In her country of origin, she had experienced physical and sexual abuse, parental abandonment, lack of formal education, and work exploitation. I marveled at her ability to escape and make her way to the United States. Once here, she had continued to work intensely—but now, of course, her resources belonged to herself and her family. In particular, she sacrificed everything for her two beloved children. Therefore, she was horrified to walk in one day and find her small daughter's nude body atop Raul's naked body. She literally broke into the room and lifted Esperanza from Raul's body, crying and yelling hysterically. Raul was drunk and put the covers over his head as Elena beat him with shoes, belts, and anything else she could get her hands on. She then told Esperanza to get dressed, and she walked her over to the emergency room, where the personnel confirmed that the child had been sexually assaulted and called the police. Elena cried so inconsolably that she was unable to say anything comforting to her daughter. Needless to say, Esperanza was terrified and confused, but she was compliant. When CPS workers arrived to talk to mother and daughter, they found Elena so distressed and unable to function that they placed Esperanza in emergency foster care—an action that went unnoticed by the mother at that moment. Esperanza, on the other hand, remained terrified until she met her foster mother, Mrs. O'Donnell. Mrs. O'Donnell was an experienced foster care worker and reassured Esperanza swiftly. Mrs. O'Donnell told me that Esperanza slept in her arms that first night.

Elena regained custody of Esperanza 3 weeks later, and it was at this point that she was referred to me.

Intake Session

Elena was severely depressed and had just had a psychiatric evaluation prior to our appointment. She told me that she would not take the prescribed medication because she did not believe in taking medication; also, she was feeling better slowly, now that the shock of what had happened was lifting. Her initial comments revealed her great grief, however. "This happened to me when I was a child," she began, "and I swore that none of my children would ever endure the pain I did." She went on to say, "I prayed to God every day for their safety, and to give me the strength to keep working and persevering." She was crying fully as she described her own "pathetic life," what she had endured, and her constant struggle to overcome what life threw her way. "I don't understand when this will end," she said with despair. "Why does everything bad happen to me? What have I done to deserve this?"

Empathizing with Elena, I tried my best to assert her amazing resiliency and to reinforce the efforts she had made for herself and her children. When we talked about Raul, she had no sympathy for him: "I hope they lock him up and throw away the keys. If I never see him again, that will be too soon." This was not a mother who expressed any ambivalence about the offender. She was clearly enraged at him for violating her trust and hurting her child. At the same time, I hadn't heard her say anything about her daughter; when I asked, she looked at me with tears in her eyes. "I can barely look at her, knowing what's happened to her." She wept uncontrollably as we talked about Esperanza. "She is an angel from God, my beautiful child. She is so good, so trusting, so sweet . . . she never asks for anything; she helps me around the house and with her brother." My heart went out to Elena. She was so distraught and felt that her life had come to an end.

I spent the last part of our 2-hour intake session trying to give Elena some sense of hope. "You have to focus on the fact that the abuse has stopped. It will not continue, and Esperanza will heal from this experience." Elena was somber when she responded, "I know, I know. I went on also, but it's never the same." I asked Elena whether she had ever been able to talk to someone, ask questions, or get some help with her own injuries. She told me that no one ever knew and that no one ever cared. I emphasized that for Esperanza things were going to be different, because this abuse was no longer a secret and we would be helping Esperanza to feel better. I also told Elena that she herself would play a big part in her daughter's recovery. Elena looked up when I said that and asked what she could do. I gave her some simple directives about nurturing and reassuring Esperanza—telling her that she was not angry with her, that she wished she had known this was going on so she could have stopped it sooner, and that both of them were going to get help to feel better. Elena repeated these messages in her own words and felt anxious to be of help to Esperanza. I remained mystified by the fact that no one had talked to the mother about how to approach her daughter, and I later discovered that I was the first Spanish-speaking person she had encountered.

I referred Elena to a Spanish-speaking colleague in my office who could see her during the day, so that she didn't have to miss work or feel overwhelmed by the demands of multiple therapy appointments in addition to court appointments. I arranged transportation through the county for Esperanza's after-school appointments.

Initial Sessions with Esperanza

Esperanza was a petite, shy, soft-spoken child. It took me a while to understand her when she spoke; she mumbled, almost literally under her breath. She entered the play therapy office, sat on the couch, folded her hands on her lap, and looked down. I told her my name; explained that I had met her mom, who had told me that Raul had hurt her private parts; and emphasized that although she had lived with another family for a while, now she was home with her mother. She nodded her head. I asked her what her mother had told her about coming to see me, and she said,

"Nothing." I told her that I saw children who had been hurt like she had, in her private parts. I also told her that she would come see me once a week, and my job was to get to know her and see if there was anything I could do to help her understand what happened to her or how she felt. Esperanza nodded again.

Then I asked Esperanza to follow me to the part of the room with the play therapy equipment, and I showed her around. She concentrated her attention on the dollhouse and began to put two babies in a toy playpen. She put a male doll on a bed and placed alcohol and beer bottles next to him. She then found a mother doll and placed her outside the dollhouse, knocking on the door. Thus began Esperanza's primary play for the first month. Meanwhile, Elena continued in therapy with my colleague and began to feel less depressed and more optimistic about her daughter's recovery. Elena reported to her therapist that her daughter had stopped having nightmares, was eating better, and seemed to be getting back to normal. The mother also specified that Esperanza felt much better in her own home and her own bed; she noted that the separation between them had been quite stressful.

Esperanza's play was quite repetitive and somewhat flat. She set up the same scenarios: Her mother was "out," her stepfather was drinking, and she and her brother were playing together. Her other scenario was that of the stepfather bathing her and getting into the bathtub with her. During this time, Esperanza would sit back, cover the bathtub with a piece of cloth, and then go play with something else. Aside from the dollhouse activity, the rest of her play seemed more generic—for example, combing a doll's hair, or using lots of mixed paints to create a picture. Of course, I noted that the combing of the doll's hair allowed her to be nurturing, and that the mixing of the paints somehow seemed to suggest her own emotional state—that is, being mixed up.

During Esperanza's play, I narrated what she did without interpretation. Esperanza listened as I did this and did not volunteer any information. When I asked a direct question about how the brother and sister felt—for example, when the mom left or came home—she was unresponsive. The other very apparent aspect of Esperanza's play was how affectively constricted she was while she played. The only exception to this was that the mixing of paints might have allowed her to be more expansive—that is, to release some affect while making large circles and adding colors with abandon.

After 2 months, Esperanza seemed "stuck" in many ways. She still spoke too quietly and rarely laughed. Elena reported that her daughter was "better," but that she was still somewhat clingy, was afraid to go outside to play, looked as if she was daydreaming from time to time, and from time to time appeared angry at her brother (striking him without any provocation). I felt it was now important to address the abuse more directly, since Esperanza's play had not allowed for sufficient movement away from the traumatic experience.

Subsequent Sessions

I told Esperanza that we were going to change what we did in our meetings. Part of the time Esperanza could do "free play" as she had before, and part of the time she and I would do some special work about her sexual abuse (I told her that this was the name for what Raul had done to her when he touched and hurt private parts of her body). I then began some TF-CBT interventions described as effective with sexually abused children (Cohen et al., 2000).

Gradual Exposure

In gradual exposure, children are encouraged to address traumatic material progressively, so that the child can tolerate and/or express more affect over time. In addition, gradual exposure allows for experiences of mastery that can result from feeling more control over the traumatic memory. Esperanza had utilized play to begin the gradual exposure process: She had chosen toy miniatures to represent her mother, stepfather, and brother; she had selected the dollhouse, which represented her family environment; she had revealed in her play that her stepfather drank and slept while she and her brother played together; and she had placed herself and her brother in a playpen, perhaps hoping to show some protection that was not afforded to her. Although the play seemed promising, it had become flat and restrained, and it did not seem to provide Esperanza with sufficient processing opportunities. She remained unresponsive to my attempts to help her expand, move, or create energy in her posttraumatic play (see Chapter Seven).

I was interested in determining whether Esperanza could tell me more about her home life—specifically, about some other traumatic event that we could explore together. In gradual exposure, it is customary to begin by helping children describe relatively less upsetting experiences. I thought I might ask about the stepfather's alcoholism, so I asked Esperanza to make a picture of her family. She was unable to complete this drawing task, so I thought it best to change media. I asked Esperanza to get the dolls from the dollhouse and put them inside the sand tray. Up to this point, she had been uninterested in playing the sand tray. She brought over the mother and stepfather dolls, the playpen with the brother and sister, and the beer and wine bottles. She placed the beer and wine bottles next to the stepfather. I asked Esperanza to tell me about the bottles.

THERAPIST: What are these?

ESPERANZA: (*Softly*) Beer.

THERAPIST: Oh, beer. Who drinks the beer?

ESPERANZA: Raul does. [This was the first time she had muttered his name.]

THERAPIST: Oh, Raul drinks the beer. (*Esperanza nods*) What happens when Raul drinks the beer?

ESPERANZA: He gets mean and yells at me and my brother.

THERAPIST: So Raul yells at you and your brother.

ESPERANZA: Yeah, he's mean.

THERAPIST: What do you and your brother do when Raul yells at you?

ESPERANZA: We go and hide under the bed.

THERAPIST: Wow, you and your brother found a place to hide from him.

ESPERANZA: Yes.

THERAPIST: What's it like to be under the bed with your brother?

ESPERANZA: It's okay. He can't find us sometimes.

THERAPIST: So sometimes he finds you and sometimes he doesn't?

ESPERANZA: That's right, sometimes he falls asleep.

THERAPIST: I see, so sometimes he falls asleep and sometimes he finds you.

ESPERANZA: Yes. (*Pause*) I want to play now.

Esperanza was on her way to verbalizing distressing experiences. I took a picture of the sand tray and reviewed it with her in subsequent sessions, as Esperanza recalled more and more experiences with her volatile, alcoholic, threatening stepfather. During these sessions, Esperanza began to show signs of anxiety, and I moved to teaching her about relaxation and managing her distress.

Relaxation and Breathing Techniques

Since physical relaxation often contributes to stress reduction, I read a book with Esperanza called *Cool Cats, Calm Kids* (Williams, 1996). This little book encourages children to mimic cats as they hiss, roll into a ball, and do other stretching and contracting exercises. Esperanza even smiled a little as she watched me do the exercises in the book. She wasn't willing to do them herself in the office, but she said she would do them with her mom at home. The book is in English, so I called Elena and told her about the book; I asked her simply to follow the cat pictures, and Esperanza would explain the rest. Sure enough, Esperanza and her mother had fun learning these relaxation exercises, and Elena reported great success with them. Esperanza responded so well to this book that I bought her and her mother cat masks, and they often wore them as they acted out the pictures in the relaxation book.

Thought Stopping

Thought stopping allows a child to interrupt distressing thoughts in a variety of ways. I encouraged Esperanza to think about a time she felt afraid. She identified the last time she felt this way, and I asked her to think about it and to stop thinking about it when the timer went off. I set the timer for 10 seconds, and when it went off, I checked to see if she had stopped thinking about feeling afraid. Esperanza learned this very quickly, and then I asked her to stop thinking when I said "Stop." Next, we traded places, and she instructed me to stop. Finally, I had her show this game to her mother, and she was able to do so at home. Once Esperanza had learned to stop the distressing thought, I asked her to think about something really nice that could take the place of a feeling she wanted to stop. She remembered a birthday party she had enjoyed when she was 5. She especially liked the fact that it consisted of just her mother, herself, her brother, and two of her cousins (i.e., the stepfather was not present). She remembered the balloons, the games they played, the food they ate, and her presents. I asked her to draw a picture of the party and she did so. I then asked her to practice stopping a thought she didn't want, and instead to remember this happy event, which could take the place of the scary or difficult thing. I also asked her to draw a picture of something scary. Kendall (1992) provides a workbook for helping children address this important concept of stopping, thinking, and establishing self-control.

Shelby (1997) has designed what she calls the "experiential mastery technique," in which children are asked to draw a picture of whatever frightens them most, are encouraged to express their feelings about their drawings, and are then instructed to do whatever they wish to their drawings that might make them feel better. Shelby has researched this technique as a crisis intervention tool with young children, and it is reminiscent of Pynoos and Eth's (1986) structured child interview. A variation of this technique utilizes miniatures in or out of a sand tray to allow children to set up a scenario that they can then move, hold, throw, bury, or otherwise manage. Some children are not positively disposed toward drawings, may feel unable or unwilling to create representational art, and may respond much more easily to a constructive strategy such as creating a (literal) scenario in a sand tray. Esperanza made her scary picture (of her stepfather coming in her bedroom door) and cut it up into little pieces she threw in the wastebasket. "You threw the cut-up picture of him in the trash," I noted. "What would you like to say to that picture?" "Be gone," she said twice, the second time in a big voice.

In addition to these specific strategies, I showed Esperanza a few videotapes: *Three Kinds of Touches* (Pennsylvania Coalition against Rape, n.d.), *Break the Silence* (Shapiro, 1994), and *Tell 'Em How You Feel* (J. Gary Mitchell Film Company, 1995). Slowly but surely, Esperanza was able to talk openly about the sexual abuse, her feelings about her stepfather, and her worries in general about her mother and the fact that she worked so much.

Cognitive Processing

Once details of the abuse become available for discussion, it is possible to identify children's misperceptions or cognitive errors, including self-blame, guilt, or extensive mistrust of adult caretakers who are of the same gender as the offender. Cohen et al. (2000) note three steps for correcting cognitive distortions: identification of children's current cognitions; evaluation of children's reasoning for distorted cognitions; and replacement of the cognitive distortions with accurate cognitions. In my experience, this takes time and needs to be accomplished over time. Sometimes children claim to understand something differently, but later on it's discovered that the same nagging cognitive distortion reappears. I think it's best for children to hear clear and concise messages in lots of different ways (e.g., in diverse therapy formats, by watching videotapes, or by reading books), and I made sure that Esperanza got these message as I worked with her.

Kendall and Braswell (1993) suggest additional strategies that can be useful with sexually abused children. These include problem-solving approaches (teaching children cognitive strategies for interpersonal problem solving); self-instructional training (self-directed statements that provide thinking strategies for children); behavioral contingencies (rewards); modeling (demonstrating behaviors to be learned by a child client); affective education (identifying emotions in self and others, and understanding the connection between emotions and behaviors); and role-play exercises (performance enhancement through practice).

Kolko and Swenson (2002) likewise suggest targeting thinking, doing, and feeling in their work with physically abused children. Since many sexually abused children often experience other forms of abuse (direct violence or witnessing domestic violence, as well as emotional abuse or neglect), their interventions are also useful. They help children identify and express feelings, learn how to relax (control their breathing, relax their muscles, use guided imagery), teach anger management (addressing aggression, power, and pride), help them cope with difficult emotions or situations, identify social supports and encourage their use by children, and utilize positive social skills. Many of these skills are taught through demonstration, rehearsal, and role plays with therapist and others, as well as instructional activities.

Creating Narratives

Another important TF-CBT strategy is the creation of a narrative about the abuse experience. This may be accomplished in a different manner, but it is an equally important component of TF-PT. By allowing children to use play and reconstruct literal aspects of their experience, as when Esperanza put her brothers, stepfather, and mother in the dollhouse, I can begin to model a narration. For example, I described what I saw: "I see that your stepdad is on the bed and he has many beer bottles next to the bed. It seems that your mom isn't home, and you and your brother are playing in the playpen." (I thought this was interesting since she was clearly too old to be inside the playpen but may have signified her wish to be more protected.) I also commented that the mother was knocking on the door and I wondered what was going on. "He told me not to answer the door no matter what. When he's sleeping, he wants us to be quiet and not answer the door." I repeated the sequence again. "Oh, I see, your stepdad has been drinking and now he's asleep, mom is trying to get in the house and he won't answer the door, and you and your brother are trying to be quiet and doing what the grownup has told you to do." I then asked, "How does that little girl feel in the playpen with her brother?" "She's scared. She wants her mom to come in and help her and she wants to be very quiet so that he stays asleep. I don't want him to wake up." "And what happens when he wakes up?" "Then he takes me to the bed . . . "

We slowly explored her thoughts, her feelings, and her behavior, but we did it through the use of miniatures that allowed Esperanza the safety and distance that she needed (at that moment) in order to begin to understand the experience. In this way, accurate narratives are modeled that children can then experience as organized, accurate expressions of events that occurred in their lives.

Termination

Once Esperanza had processed the abuse, and was able to understand that her stepfather had done something wrong and was being punished for it, she and her mother and brother attended four family therapy sessions in which we reviewed what had happened, examined how everyone felt about it, and discussed current concerns. Esperanza wanted to know how old she would be when her stepfather got out of jail; her mother responded that she would be a young woman, and that Raul would be sent to his country of origin, so she did not have to worry about his hurting her again. Elena then told Esperanza that she understood why she hadn't told her sooner about what was going on, and encouraged both children to tell her whenever anyone was hurting them, even if they knew the person or the person was a member of the family.

Esperanza had one persistent concern: She wondered whether her stepfather had been mean to her because she was bad. Apparently Raul had told her that she was a bad girl, and that her mother worked outside the home because she didn't like to be around her. Elena reassured Esperanza that her stepfather had said these things to trick her, and that she loved and liked both her children very much, but it was impossible to take care of them unless she worked very hard to make money. Esperanza listened to her mother intently and seemed to understand what Elena was telling her, but her self-doubt reappeared over time. Because of this concern, I referred Esperanza for a girls' group where she could meet other children who had been abused. I knew one other child in the group who had exactly the same worry as Esperanza, and I believed it would be helpful for them to meet and share their feelings. Esperanza truly flourished in the girls' group, and whenever I saw her in the waiting room, she would run over and give me a big hug, after asking for permission.

SUMMARY

Deblinger and Heflin's (1996) model of CBT, and Cohen et al.'s (2000) TF-CBT, are very well researched and at this time appear to be the evidence-based treatments of choice for work with sexually abused children and their families. Both utilize strategies such as gradual exposure, cognitive processing and reframing, stress management, and parental treatment. This type of therapy is directive by definition and encourages children to remember, describe, and discuss children's sexual abuse in a straightforward way. Unfortunately, not all young sexually abused children will respond to these approaches and will remain deftly resistant, dissociated, in denial, and unable or unwilling to engage in direct cognitive and verbal processing of their abuse, at least initially. Many of the specific strategies employed by CBT and TF-CBT clinicians include the use of art, puppets, books, or movies during the gradual exposure phase. My own belief is that children can utilize their natural posttraumatic play to accomplish gradual exposure and sometimes can do therapeutic processing (including cognitive processing) in this fashion.

The current trend in mental health is challenging clinicians to do treatment outcome studies in order to identify the most useful approaches for sexually abused children. In fact, Saunders, Berliner, and Hanson (2003) have evaluated current treatments and rated them on the basis of their empirical support. This material is useful in helping consumers, therapists, and others choose effective treatment strategies and avoid therapies that might range from ineffective to downright dangerous. Saunders et al. (2003) warn that their recommendations are based on evolving information in a relatively new field of study.

Too often, child therapists take an "either–or" stance when defining their theoretical positions. This frequently occurs because of apparent disparities between approaches, rigid applications, or personal commitment to practicing in pure adherence to one model or another. Such polarized thinking seems short-sighted and inflexible, however. I suggest approaching each individual child with a truly open stance, and providing services that are best suited to that child's specific learning style, defensive mechanisms, gender, culture, and developmental age and stage.

6

Family Therapy and Family Play Therapy

Child abuse can occur either within or outside the immediate family. In my opinion, abuse (especially sexual abuse) that occurs inside the home has greater complexities for children and their immediate and extended families, because of the mixed feelings that arise toward trusted family members who are suspected of abuse and the relational issues that are compromised (dependency, trust, family loyalty, etc.).

Since the early 1970s, professionals have been concerned with detection, reporting, and intervention in cases of child maltreatment in general and child sexual abuse in particular. When services specific to sexual abuse emerged throughout the country, the number of referrals were unexpected and staggering. Mental health professionals, social workers, investigators, and medical personnel have scurried to meet the ever-growing demand for specialized services in this area—specialized because of their complexity, which requires coordination among treating, protective, legal, and medical agencies.

As described in Chapter Two and mentioned throughout this book, mental health professionals working with child sexual abuse cases must be prepared to work within larger systems: familial, medical, community, legal, and those set up to protect children at risk. In addition, mental health professionals have the difficult challenge of working with families in crisis that are court-mandated to obtain treatment and are often resistant to outside interventions. Even when families voluntarily seek out mental health services, they do so with trepidation and confusion about what will be helpful in the long run. Working with families after a sexual abuse crisis is therefore multifaceted and demanding work. In addition, initial referrals are typically made for abused children, and although adults may view therapy as necessary for the children, they may resist the need for family work.

SETTING THE STAGE FOR SYSTEMIC WORK

Referral and Intake Evaluation

When a child is referred to the ACTS program, we make an initial intake appointment with one or both parents or other caretakers, as described in Chapter Two. The intake appointment is important for collecting pre-disclosure information about the child; the type and context of disclosure; the child's symptoms (if any); current social environment; and parental or caretaker observations, concerns, or questions. We also gather data about general family functioning; family dynamics that might contribute to the child's improvement or deterioration; and the parents' caretakers' willingness and ability to be of assistance to the child. In particular, because of our integrated approach and focus on children's safety, our evaluation of parents includes assessing the following: their initial and current reactions to their child's disclosure; their initial and current reactions toward the person who allegedly abused their child; and their perceptions of how and why the abuse occurred.

Initial and Current Reactions to Disclosure

Over time, it has become clear that parents will have a broad range of reactions to a child's disclosure of sexual abuse. What is inevitable is that they suffer considerable distress (Kelley, 1990). There can be expectable shock and horror at first, and parents may make statements in this context that make absolute sense—for example, "I can't believe that this could have happened." Unfortunately, if these statements are taken literally, parents can be seen as nonprotective when in fact they are reacting in an understandable way to hearing facts that appear incredible.

After the initial shock wears off, parents usually begin to consider the disclosure of sexual abuse a little more calmly. In fact, they may reevaluate their recent past in the light of this information and may find themselves piecing together scenarios that seemed innocuous prior to the disclosure. This cognitive reevaluation can elicit a broad range of reactions, including feelings of disgust, fear, sadness, betrayal, and anger. These feelings can vary from low to high intensity and seem to produce a roller-coaster effect that can disorient and destabilize even the most functional individuals. When parents of sexually abused children were themselves abused as children, a rapid succession of difficult thoughts and memories can also surface swiftly, causing further stress and debilitation or mobilizing more profound feelings of guilt for not protecting their children.

Parents who have their own history of sexual abuse appear to have one of two consistent responses to possible sexual abuse: They are either hyper- or hypovigilant to signs and symptoms of such abuse. That is, some of these parents are overly concerned with the possible occurrence of child sexual abuse, and their narrow and anxious focus on it may cause them to misinterpret or exaggerate facts. Conversely, other parents with unresolved trauma in their histories can fail to recognize clues of abuse (or fail to act on them when they do detect them), because they are uncertain about how to proceed, because they were not protected as children, or because emotions surface that are paralyzing or bewildering.

Eventually, parents seem to settle into making the protection and safety of their children their top priorities, and accepting the facts that have been revealed. This is not an immediate, abrupt event, but rather a gradual process that seems to gain momentum as parents acquire knowledge, identify and express their emotions, and receive external support. Regrettably, expecting parents to make speedy shifts in their thinking without regard to their emotional upheaval can guide the activities of CPS personnel, who may remove children from their parents' care when parents are viewed as nonprotective or unresponsive. Obviously, there are occasions that warrant instantaneous removals of children because they are being endangered by neglectful or abusive parents, but there are also occasions that require careful consideration of parents' normative initial expressions of disbelief. There are also more rare instances in which parents turn on children, accusing them of wrongdoing (seduction of adults) or abandoning them in favor of spouses or partners. Fortunately, the majority of nonoffending parents are supportive—and such support has been shown to be critical in a child's successful recovery (see "Goals of Family Treatment," below).

Initial and Current Reactions to Alleged Offenders

When intrafamilial child sexual abuse occurs, the nonoffending parent (usually the mother, as noted in Chapter Three) can have one reality and one set of emotions on one day, and be confronted with a new reality and set of emotions on the next day. I have often witnessed mothers struggling with their split loyalties, in spite of the fact that they love and want to protect their children. Many mothers have been in couple relationships that they viewed as significant or emotionally nurturing. They now have to adjust to what they perceive as the ultimate betrayal by their spouses or partners, and it's often a painful, long process that cannot be rushed. I find it useful to have open dialogues with mothers that suspend judgment and allow them to consider a wide range of responses.

Other mothers are in less conflictual situations, because their intimate relationships have been difficult or unrewarding for a long time. For these mothers, an abuse disclosure seems to tip the scales, and it's possible (even likely) that it is the proverbial last straw in a long list of injuries.

As mentioned in the preceding section, the reactions that develop over time are more telling than those that occur immediately.

Parental Understanding of How and Why Abuse Occurred

Trepper and Barrett (1989) have described four types of parental denial in child sexual abuse: denial of facts, denial of awareness, denial of responsibility, and denial of impact. I find this description accurate, in that parents may agree to the facts a child discloses, but still disagree with the abuser's motive, intent, or impact. In other words, during work with families of sexually abused children, it's critical to ensure that denial is confronted on all levels.

As parents—particularly nonoffending mothers in intrafamilial cases—struggle to understand their situation, various thoughts may be entertained. Mothers may rationalize by stating that their spouses or partners did not understand what they were doing because they were drunk; that they only did it once by accident; that they have already confessed and promised never to do it again; or that their children appear to be healthy and happy. Mothers might also believe that their spouses or partners have found religion, have sobered up, have realized the error of their ways, or have made revelations of their own histories of abuse. Men who abuse children, especially when they are arrested, charged, or imprisoned, tend to want to shift responsibility to someone or something else. Sometimes they identify the children as seductive, as compliant, or even as active participants. It is imperative for mothers to clarify how and why the abuse occurred. Many will need to be told that adults who abuse are seductive, initiate sex (whereas children may be initiating requests for affection), and often threaten children into silence. When youngsters are older, mothers seem to be very concerned with the fact that their children may not have told them about the abuse as soon as it happened.

There are several roadblocks in parental understanding that seem to appear with regularity: (1) the fact that children may disclose the abuse long after it has occurred; (2) the fact that abused children can have a range of emotions toward abusers who are parents or parent figures (e.g., feelings of sadness or loss, or an expressed desire to see them); and (3) the belief that touching or fondling may not constitute actual sexual abuse (some parents may define only penetration as true sexual abuse). All these factors need to be explored and clarified.

Educating Parents about the Multidisciplinary Process

Parents need to understand the process set into motion with a child's disclosure, particularly the various agencies, roles, and procedures that may be involved. Numerous types of professionals may come into contact with families during child sexual abuse investigation, assessment, treatment, and legal procedures. Providing information about this process and these professionals is one of the most helpful things that we can do, and it requires our own familiarity with the larger system.

I have found it useful to inform parents about the members of their helping team; to list agencies (and acronyms for those agencies); and to discuss the range of services and activities that they may encounter. Parents can be overwhelmed with the number of services they are expected to access and utilize, as well as the amount of personal information that may be requested. It's important to coordinate services in an effort to be of true assistance.

Obtaining Releases for Exchange of Information

Often clients are mandated to receive services by court order. In these circumstances, the confidentiality privilege is a moot issue, and information will be exchanged freely between the court system and its representatives and the mental health system. At the same time, since parents can often experience a sense of disempowerment when they are mandated to attend therapy or when their children are removed from their care, it is a useful clinical strategy to ask parents to give their permission to exchange information with the other members of the professional team, and to review with parents the limits of confidentiality.

The limits of confidentiality are defined by statutory duties to report certain situations. Mental health professionals are required by law to report suspected or actual child abuse and neglect, homicide, and elder abuse. Ethical responsibilities to act on behalf of suicidal clients are delineated in most codes of professional conduct.

Reviewing confidentiality privileges and allowing clients to give their permission by signature about the type and range of communications are necessary with all parents and older children. This process is absolutely critical in court-mandated cases, however, since it affords clinicians an opportunity to be viewed as trustworthy and increases the potential to form a good therapeutic alliance—a delicate issue when parents are not choosing to attend therapy voluntarily. In addition, it's clinically useful to specify what information will be shared. A good rule of thumb is to share information about attendance and cooperation. Lastly, therapists are advised to discuss information they will share, to allow clients to read some letters written to professionals (and make suggestions), or to let them listen in on some conversations with members of the professional team. Again, these activities are designed to build trust between therapists and clients, and may be particularly helpful in cases of court-mandated clients.

CHALLENGES IN FAMILY WORK

The Tendency to Over- or Underprotect the Family System

Countertransference is a powerful variable in the treatment of sexually abused children and their families. Commonly understood as the *negative* thoughts, feelings, and reactions that we therapists experience when working with clients, countertransference responses can be powerful determinants of clinical activity.[1] In sexual abuse cases, we often encounter families in crisis (which may elicit clinical urgency); multiproblem families (in which specific acts of abuse are just one family stressor); children who are removed from parents in despair; children who have mixed loyalties toward their abusers; and children who may assume that nonoffending parents will be angry at them or will not believe them (two common beliefs of abused children).

Over the years, I have noticed that professionals working on the same case may exhibit polarized responses. For example, it is not unusual for one professional to take on the role of advocate, defending all actions that a nonoffending parent takes, while other professionals may view the case in a much more punitive way. The best clinical leverage is established by being balanced in our responses to children and their families—neither condemning parents for wrongdoing, nor excusing or ignoring obvious maltreatment of children. Children's safety is our greatest concern, and acting in their best interests means that we clinicians must help to decrease family risk factors and assist in building family strengths.

---

[1] Countertransference responses need not be negative; they can be any of a broad range of responses that can affect clinical judgment in a positive or negative way. It's useful to be aware that most clinicians working with sexual abuse have strong countertransferential responses, and that attending to these is necessary to prevent burnout.

Persistent Patterns of Secrecy

In-home child sexual abuse tends to occur in families where secrecy contributes greatly to the establishment and maintenance of dysfunctional family dynamics. In order for such abuse to occur, as Finkelhor (1984) noted, family disinhibitors have to be overcome. The person who is abusing a child manages to secure the child's secrecy; the nonoffending parent does not recognize or respond to cues of family danger; and other family members remain unaware of what is occurring. There are innumerable reasons why children don't immediately break their secrecy about in-home child sexual abuse, and, likewise, multiple reasons why siblings and other family members may not recognize or acknowledge the presence of such abuse. Families are therefore likely to continue in darkness for long periods of time, and this can do untold harm to abused children. This tendency toward secrecy, moreover, can persist in other ways, indicating a habitual reliance on "circling the wagons" when in danger. Families can view external management of their lives as intrusive or threatening; they may come to feel that they have to manipulate the truth or report only partial truths, in an effort to move through the perceived demands placed on them by protective agencies. The tendency toward secrecy, coupled with resistance due to fear or anger, can become a barrier to treatment progress and needs to be explored immediately.

Multigenerational Patterns of Child Maltreatment

Not surprisingly, many parents of abused children have their own painful histories of childhood abuse. In some families, maltreatment in general or sexual abuse in particular has actually become the "norm," due to a lack of acknowledgment, disclosure, protective intervention, or any specific action on behalf of children by their parents or caretakers. The web spun by denial and silence can be intense and all-encompassing. I typically construct genograms during intake appointments (McGoldrick & Gerson, 1985), to get an overview of family issues (troubled relationships, problems, deaths, illnesses, violence, abuse, etc.), and I have found in doing so that sexual abuse is a familiar, repetitive event in many families. Indeed, I have discovered that multigenerational patterns of child sexual abuse are the rule rather than the exception and bring with them a range of challenging situations. Most important is that because there has been no intervention or treatment, child and adult victims alike have often become confused and developed learned helplessness about their plights; the cumulative trauma can be overwhelming. Even when learned helplessness is not present, these cases can be so complex that it's difficult to get a handle on what the highest priorities for services should be as the case of Lola illustrates.

Lola was a young Central American mother whose own father had sexually abused her and her sister since she was 6 years old. She eventually became pregnant by her father and had a stillborn child. Her sister Ramona, however, gave birth to her father's child before she found a man who became her pimp but agreed to give her child his last name. Lola was also pimped by her sister's partner; she did not perceive this abuse as harmful, in that she got paid money that helped her live, and it provided her with opportunities to leave the house. After Lola had two young daughters by two of her clients, she made her way to the United States to escape her father's continuing violence and predatory sexual advances. Lola's mother had fled earlier to the United States, and although Lola knew that she was well and had since remarried and had another family, Lola did not know where or how to find her.

Lola was homeless for a while, but then she somehow ended up in a shelter in which she received some skills training: She learned to wash dishes and clothes very well and went to work in a housecleaning job with two other women. She worked so hard that she was soon making enough money to rent a small room in a house with other immigrants. Lola received help in working with immigration, and over the next 6 years she established her residency and obtained a small apartment. She also married a man who was somewhat aggressive in his manner with her, but with whom she felt a camaraderie in their goals to survive and move up in the world.

This man sexually abused Lola's daughters, however, and when Lola found out she slapped the children for not telling her sooner. The children were removed from her care. When I met with Lola, several months after the removal, she was still baffled that her children had been taken; she stated that she had given her life for them, and that her long-term goal was for them to have a different life from her own. She then went on to tell me that she had told the girls every day of their lives that men were not trustworthy and would "take their bodies if they could," and that she had begged them to let her know when and if someone ever touched them. She had even touched their privates in order to make sure the girls understood what sexual touching was (a fact that the girls disclosed to CPS and that did not help Lola's case). She had slapped them from sheer despair at hearing that her attempts to prevent her girls from being abused had failed.

Lola had been told to prepare herself for a very long set of activities prior to receiving her children back to her care. The longer it took and the more probing questions she was asked about her past, however, the more she withdrew to regroup and figure out what she needed to do to regain her girls. Lola had excellent adaptive skills, and she was very "street-smart" despite her lack of formal education. She learned that there were things she needed to keep to herself and other things she should make public. When I met her she was entangled in a web of lies and deceits, not knowing whom she could trust or how she should behave. Our treatment consisted at first of establishing enough trust so that she could tell me how she was really functioning. Once this was achieved, we were able to develop a plan that worked for her: She would discuss significant feelings with me, discuss her thinking about how to proceed, and rely on me as a go-between with designated agencies. Once she felt that someone was listening to her and was on her side, she relaxed and freely discussed those things that mattered to her. Eventually we moved into an individual treatment contract that included processing her own abuse, and later I conducted family therapy sessions with Lola and her two daughters. One of the most compelling sessions I can remember with Lola was when I asked her to put words to the slap she had given her daughters upon their disclosure. Lola did a great job of explaining her fierce desire for her children's protection and her grave disappointment when she found that her children had not escaped the painful experience of sexual abuse by a parental figure.

Realities of Economics and Culture

In many child sexual abuse cases, an unfortunate set of problems may be brought about by economic limitations as well as cultural differences. Some families, particularly immigrant families, are often struggling with change of status, a new language, and/or a demanding and unfamiliar system of employment that requires documentation of previous employment history. In cases where these factors are present and where intrafamilial abuse is the issue, a swift and immediate response to signs or clues of child sexual abuse may be compromised by mothers' economic dependency on their potentially abusive spouses or partners. Obviously, this can create situations in which children are not protected, but I have learned that this is a much more convoluted issue than it first appears. In other words, sometimes mothers are thinking about their children's long-term benefits when they are thinking about abuse. They may minimize the abuse's extent or impact in favor of the basic necessities—that is, money to keep a shelter over their children's heads or food in their stomachs. Poverty, lack of preparation, feelings of helplessness, and mistrust of or unfamiliarity with helping resources are very real and deep concerns for some of the parents we treat. In addition, some mothers are the primary breadwinners in their homes and have employers too ready to dispose of them if they begin to ask for too much time off to attend court dates, visit with their children, or the like. Finally, agencies that remove children from and then return them to their families often make demands on mothers to maintain a standard of living that may be impossible for them (e.g., a separate bedroom for each child).

Accessing Community Resources

There are myriad services designed to assist children and families. Departments of social services and many other public and private child-serving organizations are established to address a wide range of child and family needs, including homelessness, physical and mental health, and education. Within these broad categories, child protection is emphasized, and a multitude of resources have been created to facilitate concrete help for indigent or high-risk families.

Surprisingly, many families remain unaware of these potential resources or may not find it possible to turn to them for help. Barriers to access are numerous and include cumbersome requirements for documentation, perceived difficulty in obtaining services, inability to communicate with professionals in one's preferred language, and (as noted earlier) a lack of motivation to seek help outside very tight family or community boundaries. Over and over I hear parents speak of their perceptions and fears about reprisal, as well as negative rumors about the dangers of exposure to outsiders. Making our services more user-friendly and more accessible remains a critical concern that must be addressed on a daily basis. It seems essential to listen well to the experiences of our clients if we are to be of true assistance.

GOALS OF FAMILY TREATMENT

A child is usually a family's entry point into treatment, particularly in cases of actual or alleged sexual abuse. As described in Chapter Two, our initial focus is on assessing the child's general functioning and identifying his or her needs vis-à-vis the sexual abuse. However, a child can never be treated in a vacuum, and gaining an understanding of the family's functioning is a parallel function of working in the best interests of the child. Deblinger, Lippmann, and Steer (1996) have found that when parents are included in treatment, and when parents are supportive of their sexually abused children, there is significantly greater improvement in children's troubled behaviors (acting out and depression). This finding highlights the importance of working with parents. As described above, however, intrafamilial child sexual abuse tends to surface in families with some level of dysfunction, which may make treatment challenging. In my experience, families with identified cases of such abuse are vulnerable families with many stressors.

Early in our understanding of child sexual abuse, there was controversy about providing family therapy in cases of intrafamilial abuse (see Friedrich, 1990, for a description of this controversy). I think these initial concerns had to do with fears that family members would be assigned equal responsibility or blame for the occurrence of sexual abuse. I believe that responsible family therapy can address issues of child sexual abuse while also placing full responsibility for sexual exploitation of children squarely on the shoulders of the persons who have committed the crime. At the same time, mothers are often disempowered by their own histories of abuse, compromised emotional states, or lack of resources. Also, in many families in which abuse occurs, mothers seek to keep their families intact once accountability and treatment have occurred. In any case, discussions of this issue have continued since the 1970s, and several texts now suggest family therapy models in the treatment of incest or child sexual abuse in general (Johnson, 2002; Maddock & Larson, 1995; Roesler & Grosz, 1993; Trepper & Barrett, 1989). Several empirically based parent–child therapies have also been found to be successful with high-risk families (Guerney, 2003; Hembree-Kigin & McNeil, 1995). In addition, CBT and TF-CBT models are anchored in direct family work (Deblinger & Heflin, 1996; Cohen et al., 2000), as noted in Chapter Five. Finally, due to the multiple stressors and high vulnerability of high-risk families, it appears critical to focus on resiliency—that is, on identifying and expanding family strengths (Kaplan & Girard, 1994; Walsh, 1998). As Friedrich (1990) states,

> Sometimes when we see only one type of child or family, we may believe that abuse is either much more discrete in its impact or primarily very negative. It is important to recognize this variability because it reminds us again of the hopefulness that can be present even in traumatic events and that the possibility of change always exists. It also forces us to realize that there are strengths and sources of resilience in the individuals whom we see that exceed any of the curative powers that we might be able to bring to these dysfunctional families. (p. 102)

Most practitioners concur that the following goals are critical in working with families of sexually abused children:

1. Assessing family functioning in terms of strengths and vulnerabilities, and identifying high-risk factors.
2. Assessing family members' responses to the immediate crisis generated by a sexual abuse disclosure.
3. Helping family members process their thoughts and feelings regarding the sexual abuse.

4. Strengthening the parents' ability and willingness to respond appropriately to this family crisis.
5. Conducting trauma-focused work.
6. Redefining roles and responsibilities of family members.
7. Providing reunification services when appropriate.

The term *"trauma-focused* work" refers to the following: Parents will be helped to face denial in all its forms, to process their own responses to child sexual abuse (gradual exposure), to develop coping strategies, and to learn skills for helping their children and developing prevention strategies for their future.

These goals are advanced by providing traditional individual, family, and group psychotherapy. Depending on children's ages and stages of development, as well as parents' level of resistance, compliance, motivation, and cooperation, family play therapy may increase the likelihood of full participation by family members; I describe family play therapy and illustrate its use in the case illustration of the Daniels family, below. Of paramount clinical interest is increasing family members' receptivity to therapy, and consistent efforts must be made to find creative and useful approaches.

FAMILY TREATMENT PLANS AND SERVICES

Treatment plans may include a variety of conjoint services for children and their families and caretakers (including foster parents and legal guardians). Family therapy can be conducted through one person, in parent–child dyads, and with full participation from all available family members. There are two common circumstances that occur with regularity in our sexual abuse treatment program: (1) in-home sexual abuse, which may include temporary family separation, specialized services for family members with sexually abusive behaviors (see below), and reunification plans; and (2) out-of-home sexual abuse, which may or may not include a course of supportive, psychoeducational, crisis intervention, or traditional family therapy. It's important to note that in both these circumstances, children's allegations of sexual abuse tend to bring families to the attention of the legal system and social service agencies, whose investigators evaluate the context in which sexual abuse has been alleged or has occurred. These investigations can result in the detection of a variety of parallel concerns, such as neglect, lack of supervision, family violence, substance abuse problems, or other factors that might elicit concern and/or further involvement from these first-contact agency personnel.

SPECIALIZED SERVICES FOR OFFENDERS

I have written elsewhere about the unique aspects of family therapy with families in which sexual abuse occurs (Gil, 1985). The field of sex offender treatment is likewise highly specialized and replete with research and innovations. A national organization (the Association for the Treatment of Sexual Abusers, or ATSA) has successfully established a leadership role and generates high visibility as it advocates for specialized training for those professionals committed to being of assistance to children, teens, or adults who have sexually abusive behaviors. In cases of in-home child sexual abuse, our clinicians recognize the need for close collaboration with sex offender specialists; we consider ourselves to be working within an inclusive team that is focused on ensuring children's safety and strengthening and preserving the family unit whenever humanly possible.

CASE ILLUSTRATION: THE DANIELS FAMILY

Sometimes alligators are just being alligators . . .

The Daniels family, an African American family, was referred to me because of the alleged acquaintance rape of 14-year-old Sheila. Because the mother's immediate reaction was to be angry and skeptical at her daughter, Sheila and her mother agreed with CPS that Sheila would go to live with her birth father in Europe, at least to complete her high school education. Sheila had visited him every summer, had good friends near her father's home and in the local school there, and described her relationship to her father as calmer than that with her mother. Sheila's birth father had readily agreed to his daughter's living with him, his current wife, and his twin sons, approximately 7 months old.

During the initial investigation, before Sheila left for Europe, the social worker noted that the mother, Estelle, had an overtly conflictual relationship with her daughter; however, she also found Sheila a bit withdrawn and negative. In addition, the social worker noticed that Estelle was under a lot of pressure. She seemed very "stressed out" and complained that she was at her wits' end with her only son, Jackson. Mrs. Daniels was the mother of four children: Sheila, 14; Michelle, 12; Jackson, 6; and Chloe, 4.

Early Sessions with the Mother

I did an intake session with the mother after Sheila's departure, and I quickly agreed with the social services worker that Estelle was under significant stress raising four children on her own. The mother made it very clear that Sheila was not the problem. She stated, "Just trust me on this one: Whatever happened to Sheila was probably not as bad as she told people. I think she's basically where she wants to be. I talk to her every week, and she's doing just fine. I need help with the rest of this crew, especially Jackson!" Estelle added that Sheila would return for summers, and that maybe I could meet her in the future so that I could see she was "just fine."

Estelle then proceeded to tell me that Chloe, her youngest child, was the child of a recently ended marriage that the mother described as "rough." When I asked for a clearer description, she replied that she wasn't there to talk about herself; she just wanted someone to "deal with" her son, Jackson. Despite her reluctance, I took down as much information as I could in our first meeting. This included hints of relational problems with men, a history of physical abuse in her childhood, and possible domestic violence in two of her relationships. I gave Estelle a lot of support for juggling her job, a partial school schedule, and the competing demands of her four children. She spoke of them lovingly but begrudgingly, often stating that she worked so hard for them and felt that they did not appreciate how good they had it. She was spirited; had good boundaries; asked for very specific help in managing her son; and was remarkable in her intense desire to raise "decent, honest, educated children."

I described the assessment process to Estelle, and it fit very well with her expectations that I was there to help her son. I asked her to meet with me a second time, because I felt I had not gathered enough information that would prepare me to meet with Jackson. She grunted, but agreed to come back so that she could help me get the "big picture." I also told her that in the process of trying to understand the specific problems she had with Jackson, I might invite her and her other children to participate in family sessions from time to time. "Oh, Lord," she said, "that will be a circus!" I was curious about her disparaging comment and made a mental note to explore it further when I had met with Jackson.

During our second meeting, I pursued Estelle's specific complaints about Jackson. She described herself as being "fed up" with Jackson's constant back-talking and failure to comply with even the most basic house rules. She described feeling frustrated with his aggression, hyperactivity, and oppositional behavior. She seemed to single him out among her children, describing the girls as "much easier to handle." Even Sheila, whom she had described as "having issues," seemed to generate considerably less negativity than her son did. I was curious about Jackson's behaviors, and I asked the mother when they had begun. When I opened this door, Estelle opened herself up by recounting her recent history with Chloe's father, Michael.

Estelle seemed to release a lot of pent-up emotions during this narrative (and confided at the end of this second session how surprised she was by her "endless gabbing"). She described herself as going through a recent transformation, claiming disbelief and horror at how she had "allowed herself to feel dominated" by Chloe's father. They had married after a brief office romance, and Mrs. Daniels described an immediate, abrupt change in her husband following their honeymoon. "I have never seen anyone change so drastically," she revealed. "It was as if I had married one man and come home with another." She told me that Michael became moody, irritable, and intolerant of her and her children: "Everything they did drove him wild." She added, "The kids didn't know whether they were coming or going; one minute he was nice and fun; the next he would turn on them, yelling in their faces and making them go to their rooms." She expressed her guilt and shame, stating, "It was bad enough I let him treat me like a dog; I can't believe I let him behave that way with my children . . . that's something I'll regret till the day I die."

Responding to my initial question, Estelle noted that her troubles with Jackson had begun shortly after Michael began his abusive behavior toward them. "It was almost like Jackson was trying to be all bad, like his dad," she said. (She was referring to Michael, although Jackson's birth father had also been an aggressive man, as she later revealed.) "Sometimes he would put his arms on his hips, stick his chest out, and defy me to make him do something he didn't want to do." She added, "A few times, he actually said, 'You can't make me. You're just a stupid girl.' " The mother also mentioned that Jackson suddenly became very rude to his sisters, and often chased them around the house shouting at them.

At the conclusion of this second meeting with Estelle, I stated the obvious:

> "Well, it sounds like you and your family have been through a lot. I am also encouraged to hear that you and Jackson have had a more positive relationship in the past than the one you're having right now. It sounds like before Michael and you married suddenly, Jackson was having fewer problems with his behavior. It sounds like Jackson might have learned some unfortunate lessons from Michael . . . I'm not sure, of course, but I thank you so much for sharing this information, because it was important for me to know about in order to be of help to you and your family."

We agreed on a mutually convenient appointment time for Jackson, and the mother seemed motivated to return.

Conjoint Sibling Sessions

Estelle's description of Jackson had led me to brace myself for my first meeting with him (and actually to take some toys out of the play therapy office). I was pleasantly surprised to find that Jackson was a bright, presentable, coy child of 6; no trace of his "provocative manner" was discernible. After my first few sessions with him, in which he explored the room freely and interacted calmly with me, I asked his sisters Chloe and Michelle to join us for conjoint family therapy sessions. The mother usually brought her own school work to the waiting room, and she reported that it was useful to have a spare hour in which to do this work. Her two girls brought toys and seemed to entertain themselves easily. They seemed eager to see the play therapy office that their brother had described in exaggerated fashion. ("There are *not* five million toys in here!" exclaimed older sister Michelle upon entering the room.)

Early conjoint therapy sessions with the three children revealed two patterns. First, Jackson was frequently ignored by his two sisters; although he often distracted himself and played alone, he seemed to become visibly frustrated or upset when he felt that he was not allowed to join in play with them. The other consistent pattern was one of fear, anxiety, and loss. Much of the children's collective play demonstrated how much they missed their older sister and how many fears they had about "bad men," "angry men," and "mean men." Although I asked general questions about Michael, and I had told them what I knew about their family situation, they revealed little and often appeared shy or uncomfortable discussing him. Michelle had noted, "I don't like to think about him," and "I'm glad he's gone." The other children did not express an opinion either way, but there was usually a hush in the room when Michael's name was mentioned by anyone.

The children created scenarios or stories in the sand, often setting up miniatures and then acting out stories. In this active, constructive play, animals were often lurking on the outside of houses or neighborhoods, hiding from view, ready to attack. Sometimes when family members were sleeping in their beds, secret tunnels were being dug underneath the house, so that "bad creatures" might crawl inside. Michelle was definitely the initiator of most play when the three children were together, and Chloe was remarkably mature and self-sufficient for her age.

Jackson's behavior during therapy was absolutely within the typical range for his age in terms of aggression or noncompliance. He liked the fact that he could choose what to play with, and often stopped play with one toy or game after a brief time, moving to another one. When I tried to encourage more joint activities among the three siblings, Michelle and Chloe would invariably lock heads and work together, leaving Jackson to feel excluded and isolated. In response, Jackson distracted and provoked them by interfering with their play, making rude comments to them, or becoming unfocused and loud in his own activities. Jackson's behavior seemed directly related to his feeling excluded, which he perceived as a rejection and which therefore elicited emotions of helplessness and anger.

I was left to surmise how this pattern was helped or hindered by the mother's presence, and whether the girls' apparent exclusion of their brother represented some sanction against his gender and their negative experiences with males.

These conjoint sibling sessions were quite informative and highlighted potentially problematic interactions. They also revealed these children's shared experience of living with an unpredictable, violent person; the youngsters had now internalized their worries and felt anxious about their current safety and ongoing security. I remember Chloe's once saying, "He can find us if he wants," referring to their relocation to a new home since the mother's separation from Michael and her own apparent fear that she might not be safe enough. I encouraged Chloe to tell her mother about this fear, and it led the family to make a safety plan about Michael.

After three conjoint sibling sessions, I asked Mrs. Daniels to join us in the next meeting for a family play therapy session (the rolling of her eyes was duly noted).

Family Play Therapy

Elsewhere (Gil, 1994, 2003b), I have described "family play therapy" as the convergence of two major clinical approaches: family therapy and play therapy. It simply means using a range of play (or other expressive) therapy techniques and approaches to elicit the full participation of family members (of diverse ages, developmental stages, and genders). This is done in order to uncover, address, and resolve presenting problems or underlying patterns of family dysfunction.

The interest in family play therapy is often overshadowed or compromised by patronizing or disparaging perceptions of play therapy. A highly respected colleague summed up his skepticism by asking me, "I see the play, but where is the therapy?" The field of family play therapy continues to struggle with such skepticism, and yet it has made great strides toward credibility and respectability in the last two decades. A handful of pioneers are continuing to report on their work in family play therapy, and empirical evidence for its usefulness is being undertaken and documented (Bratton, Ray, & Rhine, 2005).

Family Puppet Therapy

An early technique involving family puppet work was developed by Irwin and Malloy (1975) as an interview tool with families, and this tool is described more specifically elsewhere (Gil, 1994). It has since served as a springboard for an expanded therapeutic approach that can be used during the assessment phase or throughout treatment, once or multiple times.

Family puppet therapy is thus not limited to the interview/assessment phase, although it can be quite informative for these purposes. This type of therapy is built on an understanding of storytelling, as well as identification and use of metaphorical language. The use of puppets adds a creative, dynamic element that appears to energize families. In addition, by getting into character and endowing puppets with voices, traits, and behaviors, family members use projection to introduce areas of interest, underlying concerns, conflicts, and potential resolutions. Family puppet therapy has immeasurable potential to allow or encourage family members to communicate symbolically, decrease defenses, experience individual and collective pleasure, and develop more successful and rewarding exchanges with each other.

In family puppet therapy sessions, it is important to provide ample choices in both numbers and types of puppets. I usually bring out 20–30 puppets for family use, and I instruct family members to choose the puppets they find interesting or attractive for whatever reason. I then provide the following simple directions:

> "I'd like you to make up a story with a beginning, a middle, and an end. There are only two rules. First, you have to make up the story together (rather than tell a story that someone has read, heard, or seen on TV or in the movies). Second, you have to act out the story, rather than narrate it. I'm going to give you about 20 minutes to develop your story. Let me know when you're done, and I'll come back in to listen to your story."

Depending on the ages of participating children, they may need some role modeling.

The family members are then given a reasonable period of time in which to develop their story (20 minutes), and the therapist may leave the room, or stay in the room as a quiet observer. Another option for a clinician who has the appropriate technology is to leave the room, observe the family through a one-way mirror, and videotape both the story's development and the story as eventually told to the clinician.

During the family's creation of a story, it is interesting and informative to observe how the family organizes itself around a joint task. Many family dynamics can be documented, such as cooperation, level of encouragement and support, types of communication styles, interactional patterns (particularly family alliances), individual participation and the extent to which it·is sought or accepted by other family members, and the ability to stay focused and complete the task. It is also fruitful to note any alterations in the story between the creation and rehearsal of the story and the storytelling to the therapist.

Most families can develop and rehearse a story within 20–30 minutes.

Large families may take longer, and on occasion I have heard a family's puppet story in a subsequent session. Sometimes a discussion of what is challenging or easy about creating stories may be in order. Finally, some families end up having so much fun that the storytelling can be delayed in favor of enhanced family dynamics.

Having done literally hundreds of family puppet sessions, I assert that it is unusual for families to be unable to create a story together. In the two or three occasions I have witnessed when families could not accomplish this task, the families had a stressor that could account for the members' inability to work together (e.g., a family with a lack of biological connection; a mother who had decided to relinquish parental rights; parents who had decided to divorce but had not told their children).

When I began using family puppet therapy with the Daniels family, Jackson and his siblings were fascinated by the video camera and took turns looking through it. They also looked over and selected puppets, choosing to separate the puppets into two stacks: the ones they would use in their story, and the ones they would not. I was impressed with their organizational skills. As I gave my directions, they listened intently and asked a few clarifying questions. As soon as I left the room, Michelle took charge, allowing her visibly tired mother to sit back in a chair and relax.

The mother had a faint smile on her face as she watched her children develop the puppet story. Michelle and Chloe worked together on the story while Jackson chose his puppet, an alligator, and then seemed to acquiesce to his older sister's demands: "You don't live with us; you live in a pond. Go over there." Jackson found a large blue pillow and proceeded to make a comfortable spot for himself, separate but close to his family. "This is my pond," he said proudly.

When I observed the family's approach to completing this task, I noticed that Michelle and Chloe appeared very close and cooperative. Soon to be 5 years old, Chloe was unusually mature and task-focused for her age. Michelle solicited her sister's cooperation with a combination of persuasion and humor. This behavior was in sharp contrast to what appeared to be her marginal interest in, and sometimes even slight irritability toward, her brother. The mother seemed somewhat detached, but was responsive to the children's sporadic queries to her. After 25 minutes, Michelle asked Jackson to go and tell me that they were ready to tell their puppet story. I sat down and listened to the following story, narrated by Michelle and acted out by herself and the others:

One girl comes over to pick up another girl to go to school. The girls greet each other, the second girl kisses her mother goodbye, and off they go to school. On the way, they notice a pond, and the girl suggests to her friend that they go visit the pond. As they get close to it, an alligator jumps out and begins to snap his jaws. He bites the first girl, and they run back home. Meanwhile, the mother has been cleaning and welcomes the girls home. The girls promptly complain about the alligator in the pond who scared them. The mother asks whether they were hurt, and they say no, at which point the alligator bursts in and says, "Yeah, you were. I bit you." The mother then asks where they saw this alligator and how come they haven't been at school. The girls state that they went to school first, but "it was closed," so they went for a walk by the pond. They refocus on the scary alligator, and the mother repeats that it's important that they walk straight to school and not go off by themselves. The alligator then asks the girls to come back to the pond and play with him, and promises not to bite them again. The mother goes and punishes the alligator, and the girls get sent to bed. This is the end.

Family puppet therapy sessions can quickly become very challenging. The clinician needs to make immediate decisions about how to proceed, what to emphasize, or where to direct the family's focus. I decided first to ask Estelle to talk to the alligator. "Mrs. Mom," I stated, "I would like you to take a trip to the pond and go talk to the alligator about his biting behaviors."

"Okay," she said in a cooperative voice, "even though I'm tired from working all day, I'm going to make a trip to the pond, and girls, be sure you have done your chores when I get back here." The mother took her puppet over to the blue pillow where Jackson and the alligator were. When she got there, she asked the following questions: "Why are you so angry and hurting everybody? Is it that you don't want anyone touching you?" I was surprised by her questions, but I remembered that she had once confided to me that she found it difficult to be physically affectionate to Jackson because of his aggression. His mother's questions didn't leave Jackson much room for response; Jackson swiftly placed his alligator under the pillow. I told the mother that maybe she could try again— this time simply telling the alligator that she did not want him to bite or scare her girls, but that it was okay if they wanted to play together. Estelle turned again to Jackson (and his alligator) and said, "I just don't know why you're trying to scare and hurt those poor girls." Jackson did not respond, so I decided to grab a puppet and come into the story.

I grabbed a fish puppet and brought it near the pond. "Hello there, Mrs. Mom. I am Gunther, and I live here in this pond with Mr. Alligator. I just thought I'd let you know what I've learned about Mr. Alligator by living with him these many years." Jackson was really attentive to me and my fish puppet. "Sometimes alligators are just being alligators . . . They have big mouths and big teeth, and so people are often scared of them and stay away. Alligators have never learned how to behave because most people are scared and throw rocks at them, and basically don't understand them because they look scarier than they are." The mother then stated clearly, "Well, I know they look scary, but sometimes they don't know how scary they can be." I used my fish puppet to say, "You're right. He can look scary with his big teeth and all. But sometimes they're just doing the best they can, since they don't have any good practice in being friendly to others."

Estelle then offered, "Must be hard to be alone all the time." Jackson in his best alligator voice said, "Yeah, I just want to play . . . I want them to come play with me." His mother then used her puppet's hand to pat the alligator puppet on the head: "Okay, okay, let's make a deal . . . as long as you agree to not bite or scare the girls, I'll let them come out and play." Jackson's voice grew louder as he said, "Hooray, hooray!" Estelle took her puppet and told the girl puppets, "You can go to the pond and play with that lonely alligator, but let me know if he tries to hurt or bite you again." I would have preferred the mother to predict that the alligator would not bite or scare them again. I then took my fish puppet and whispered to the alligator puppet, "Okay then, you better decide quick what kind of game you want to play, and make sure you don't bite or scare those girls, or they won't want to come back again. This is your big chance, Mr. Alligator. You and I always have fun playing, and I know you can do it without hurting them."

The girl puppets arrived at the pond and hollered for the alligator (who was again under the blue pillow): "Mr. Alligator, Mr. Alligator, where are you? We came back to play. Our mom gave us permission." Jackson peeked out and told them, "Hi, I know what we can play." "What?" the girls asked. "Hide and seek," Jackson said with gusto. "I'll hide and you try to find me." At that point, the girls and Jackson played a couple of rounds of hide and seek. Our session time had come to an end, but since the children were having such a positive interaction, I extended the session a few minutes. Their mother spontaneously said, "Now that's more like it. See how you guys can play without problems?" Gunther came out at the last minute and said goodbye. "I gotta go now, everybody. I got to go catch dinner." Everyone waved goodbye to my fish puppet.

After listening to this story, I felt that some of my initial impressions about the family had been confirmed: The sequence of interactions among the children and their mother reinforced the problem behaviors. Jackson often felt rejected by his sisters, became resentful and aggressive, and then acted out with his siblings. They in turn complained to their mother, who became more and more intolerant of Jackson's aggression. Jackson was more often than not the recipient of negative attention, and yet seemed to long for companionship and nurturing. At the same time, Jackson also seemed invested in his aggressive role, insisting that his sisters adequately represent the alligator as biting one of them, rather than just as being scary.

I gave Estelle a copy of this videotaped story, and she told me at our next scheduled appointment that the children had watched it together at least five times during the week. "Even I've watched it twice, which is saying a lot . . . I can't believe how tired I look in that tape."

I asked Estelle what other observations she had about the family puppet therapy session, and she seemed to have given this quite a bit of thought. She repeated that she'd noticed how tired she looked; she then noted how sad Jackson looked when his sisters didn't want to play with him, and how goofy the alligator looked. "I don't know if it's your alligator or what, but it's hard to get angry at that alligator or feel too scared of him. He almost looks like an alligator pretending to be a tough guy." I inquired about the potential benefit to an alligator of looking tough, and she said, "Well, I guess that just keeps him feeling safer."

I then gave her feedback about the story, documenting the positives first. I reinforced how well they had all done in creating and rehearsing the story, and how even though it was clear how tired Estelle was, she had stayed available to her children. I also emphasized how the girls had gone out exploring together and how they had returned to the mother to inform her about their dangerous adventure. I further supported the mother's willingness to go speak to the alligator and to cut a deal that might be a win–win situation for both. Even though the mother's initial responses to the alligator in the story had been closed- rather than open-ended, she was able to readjust and follow through in a more productive way.

Estelle listened attentively, and then described the past week (since the puppet session) with great insight. She reported that she had found herself musing about the puppet story throughout the week, particularly her newfound tolerance for her son. "I think I was secretly afraid that he was just like his real dad, and every time I corrected him, I was correcting his dad. Of course, with Jackson, it worked for a short time . . . his dad never did listen." I talked with the mother for a while about how important it was for her to set good limits with Jackson about his aggressive behaviors, but I emphasized that it was equally important to empathize with his situation. In particular, I noted, it was critical for her to realize that Jackson was the only boy in a family with three girls (one currently absent) and a single mother. Jackson's birth father, as well as his stepfather, had been violent and frightening. In fact, Jackson had received a lot of modeling about male aggression, and his mother was hypersensitive to signs of aggression in him—often anticipating or expecting negative behaviors, and sometimes chastising him in order to prevent his negative acting out. I was pleased to hear the mother's reflective thoughts and supported her insight.

Estelle also reported another very useful shift in perception—specifically, that Jackson had "boy energy," which was quite different from "girl energy." When I asked her to elaborate, she noted that her girls often spent quiet time playing and liked to use pretend play. Jackson, she noted, was all movement and action, and he never seemed to relax. "The girls like to cuddle in bed with me sometimes," she added thoughtfully; "him, I can't catch and hold down long enough to give him a hug!"

Estelle also shared with me that their puppet story had occurred outdoors rather than within confines. She seemed melancholy as she remembered a time some years back, when the family seemed to have regular weekend picnics. She then reported to me that she had good news, and told me about a weekend outing that had been truly fun for everyone. "It was fun to watch Jackson run around as much as he wanted . . . He seemed happy if I just counted his laps or timed how long it took him to run around the small lake." She seemed to be acknowledging that when Jackson received positive attention, he seemed more content. Lastly, she confided that she had brought a Frisbee to the park, and that Jackson had a chance to coach both his sisters in throwing and catching.

Comments on This Use of Family Play Therapy

As you can see in this example, the use of a family play therapy technique (puppet therapy) was inviting to all family members and expanded their repertoire of communication and contact. It almost always offers a true opportunity to have a mutually beneficial interaction, void of conflict and pressure. In some cases, engaging in family play therapy immediately can signal deficits in the amount or quality of time the family spends together. Most importantly, conducting family play therapy usually allows adults (more often than children) to contemplate their situation in different ways and to consider how the play informs and shapes their responses. The types of insights reported by Estelle, the mother in this chapter's case illustration, occur more often than not and provide a springboard for further consideration and action.

In this clinical illustration, much was revealed by content and process. The family puppet therapy, as well as the conjoint sibling sessions and individual therapy sessions with the mother, consistently revealed a series of issues that had contributed to the emergence and maintenance of problem behaviors in the family. When Estelle was referred for treatment, she was under a great deal of stress, had a history of violence in intimate relationships, and was maintaining jobs both in and out of the home. Certain dynamics were occurring without her conscious understanding; in particular, Jackson's gender made him vulnerable to being seen as a potential aggressor. His mother found it easier to manage her more compliant daughters, and her behavior was inadvertently contributing to all three of them ignoring, chastising, or expelling her son. Jackson adequately perceived rejection from his family and developed resentment, which he then acted out aggressively. Once Estelle was able to see her son as a boy child with a tender heart, she was able to shift her behaviors toward him, so that Jackson immediately felt more accepted and acceptable. His mother was eventually capable of seeing him as a little boy who had unique energy, rather than a child who was destined to behave like his threatening father and stepfather.

There were other issues that were addressed in subsequent family therapy sessions, and we used family play therapy techniques intermittently throughout our work.

Family Art Evaluation

The technique of family art evaluation was developed by Kwiatkowska (1978). It consists of asking family members to make a series of pictures on easels placed in a semicircle. The pictures requested are as follows: (1) anything that comes to mind; (2) a family portrait (realistic or abstract); (3) an individual scribble; (4) a family scribble; and (5) again, a picture of anything that comes to mind. Each family member makes a total of four individual pictures, and the family together creates one picture (the family scribble). For the purposes of this chapter, I will describe the Daniels family's scribble picture, which once again aptly revealed the family's persistent problem dynamic. The scribble project also indicates how families can carry over metaphors from one medium to another.

As mentioned above, the family scribble takes place after each family member has already made three individual pictures. This fourth task invites the family to work cooperatively and create something "together, as a family." This family task allows a clinician to view the family's customary way of organizing and completing a task; it illustrates who is left out, who participates, who cooperates, how conflict is dealt with, and whether the family is generally cohesive or fragmented.

Jackson's family (Estelle, Michelle, Chloe, and Jackson himself) had completed their early pictures without incident. The family portraits (drawn as the second task) had excluded the oldest sister, except for the mother's drawing, which indicated that Sheila was on her mind (she drew little circles vertically and then created a cloud-like shape with a young girl inside). Jackson asked the identity of the girl in the cloud;

when Estelle answered that it was the children's oldest sibling, Sheila, everyone commented how much they missed her.

They each made their individual scribbles quickly and seemed interested in how it was possible to find the shapes of familiar things within a scribble. Having had individual experiences with the scribble, the family members were then asked to look at a new set of scribbles and choose which one they would use to create a picture together.

After some discussion, the mother's scribble was chosen. The family members began to draw a fruit salad, each child choosing colors to fill in the fruits—papaya, melon, pineapple, and kiwi. As the others talked about their fruits and seemed to have fun making decisions about fruit selections and colors, Jackson was excluded more and more. At first he couldn't decide which fruit to be, and then he couldn't decide on a color. He was getting tired and grumpy, and seemed to feel rejected as his mother and sisters laughed together. He chose to sit in a corner, frowning and pouting. Estelle encouraged him to join in a few times, but then she apparently forgot about him.

The picture was nearly completed when Jackson "walked" on his knees over to the bottom of the easel, and with the ever-so-light pressure of a green crayon, started to draw a small figure in the bottom left-hand corner. His mother and sisters inquired vigorously about what Jackson was making, and why he wasn't making a fruit for the fruit salad. Finally, in a quiet voice, Jackson stated, "I am the alligator, coming for dinner." The mother and sisters reacted in unison: "Oh, no! The alligator can't come to dinner . . . we're having fruit, and they don't eat fruit." Jackson protested mildly that he did like fruit and he was hungry for dinner, but his voice was barely heard over their protestations. Jackson then placed an eyeball on the alligator in such a way to indicate that the alligator, initially entering the picture from the corner, was now exiting the picture at the corner. Jackson then retreated to the corner, where he remained for the rest of the session, unwilling to complete the last picture of the family art evaluation. Clearly, the same dynamic seen in the puppet play had occurred in the brief time it took to make the family scribble: Jackson could not find a way to fit into the otherwise all-female family; the closer they became, the more excluded he felt; he then chose his familiar alter ego, the alligator (a symbol of aggression) to make his way into the family picture; the family rejected the alligator and misinterpreted his wish to join the family at the dinner table, instead viewing the alligator's arrival (or participation) as a threat; Jackson then withdrew, and eventually became aggressive and uncooperative.

When the family members and I reviewed all the drawings, we had a therapeutic conversation about the fruit salad, and what they had noticed about how things went during the development of the fruit salad. Michelle noted that Jackson had been "a brat," and I took that opportunity to review how things had actually developed. I asked Michelle to stop the tape and rewind to what it was like before her brother had been what she called "a brat." As we did this exercise, the mother and Michelle noted that they had gotten very involved with their art project, and maybe that had made Jackson feel left out. We then talked about how people express their feeling of being left out, and they described lots of behaviors—some funny, some odd. Estelle once again was able to understand her son's need to be part of the family, and how easy it was to fall into a pattern of rejecting him because he had a more "energetic and curious" personality. "We all chose our fruits right away," she noted. "He couldn't make up his mind and kept coming up with goofy suggestions. We should have waited until he stopped." The mother then once again announced her intent to show Jackson that he was an important part of the family, and seemed to gain quite a bit of insight about the process they had undertaken.

Family Sand Therapy

Therapy proceeded well; I began seeing Jackson less frequently on a one-to-one basis, and more as part of a larger family unit. I used conjoint whole-family and sibling sessions until Jackson and his sisters began to find common ground, and to respect and value each other's differences. Toward the end of treatment, I asked the family once again to undertake a joint family project: a family sand tray. Jackson and his sisters were familiar with the sand tray and looked forward to showing their mother what to do.

The creation of the family sand tray was a sign of this family's improvement and greater cohesion. In the bottom right-hand corner, a beach scene emerged—the children loved excursions to the beach, and had drawn many pictures of themselves at the ocean. In this scene, everyone in the family was included: the mother, Jackson, and his sisters. Everyone was swimming in protected waters, "with no sharks," and there were umbrellas in case the sun got too hot.

In the upper left-hand corner, Jackson placed a building, with a motorcycle and a fast car outside. This was the alligator's house, and the alligator was outside, "hanging out and looking around." Jackson then announced: "The people on the beach are safe, because there's a guard that makes sure that the alligator doesn't go too far and scare people." Jackson seemed to be indicating that he had learned ways of controlling his aggressive impulses. He also seemed to be suggesting that he felt himself to be more a part of his family, and perhaps had realized that his aggression did not serve him well.

Michelle chose a different message altogether: She put a bride and groom getting married in front of a church. Directly behind the bride and groom was a cemetery—perhaps indicating Estelle and Michael's (or Estelle and her birth father's) "dead" marriage, or her pessimism about marital success.

Chloe placed birds' nests in the trees, and a dog family shaded under a big tree.

Everyone participated in and felt proud of their collective product. The mother smiled as she looked at the beach scene, reminiscing about good times they had had in the past. I had to take four pictures of the completed sand tray, since everyone insisted on having his or her own to take home.

Later Sessions and Termination

We also did recreational therapy in some later sessions. This seemed to be a favorite activity of Jackson's: in these sessions, he relished the opportunity to teach his sisters some athletic skills, and they were interested and willing students.[2]

Estelle and I met monthly to discuss parenting issues, as well as how to present information to her children about separation and divorce. She read a book to the children, *Dinosaurs Divorce* (Brown & Brown, 1988), and the children were better able to talk about their loss. I counseled the mother that even though the children's father and stepfather had been abusive, it is not uncommon for children to have loving feelings toward an absent parent. I gave her the concept that she (and they) could absolutely condemn violent behavior and still feel empathy towards the person. This concept of separating the behavior from the person became useful when we were discussing Jackson's aggression as well.

I was able to meet Estelle's oldest child when she came home for the summer. When Sheila reentered the family system, the children made a quick adjustment: Michelle shared her "oldest child" status with Sheila,

---

[2] Abused children sometimes carry tension and stress in their bodies and can have contracted muscles, restricted breathing patterns, and lack of fluidity in their movements—they can appear "stiff" and uncomfortable in their bodies. Often they have experienced pain and discomfort in their bodies either due to physical violence, boundary violations, or lack of appropriate hygiene or nutrition. They can also develop somatic complaints such as stomachaches, headaches, and hypersensitivity to injury. Because of this, it may be helpful to encourage a broad range of physical activity, such as dancing, running, movement, gymnastics, and team sports like basketball or softball. These recreational activities allow children to explore their bodies, release constricted energy, and experience a sense of well-being and enjoyment.

and Jackson and Chloe shared more activities as the two older girls got reacquainted and shared clothes, makeup, and boy stories. The mother asked me to see Sheila individually to discuss her allegation of date rape and to make sure she was doing all right. I met with Sheila for a while, and then met with the mother and daughter together to discuss the past—especially the mother's reactions upon hearing the disclosure— and to reestablish open lines of communication about this and other topics. Estelle was patient and understanding with Sheila; in turn, Sheila explained that her abuse had been experienced less as a trauma and more as an opportunity to make an early departure to live with her father abroad. At one point the mother noted, "I knew it, I knew it. I knew you were exaggerating the whole thing to get what you wanted." Sheila apologized and told her mother she loved her, but she felt very secure in her relationship to her, unlike the relationship with her father. "I just wanted to go live with Dad and get to know him better . . . I felt like he had other kids now, and he was gonna love them better." Estelle hugged her daughter, seemingly understanding Sheila's need for security in her relationship to her father.

SUMMARY

Working with child maltreatment—especially child sexual abuse—in families is complex and challenging. By necessity, clinicians are required to operate within professional teams, and their roles are often expanded to include advocacy and court testimony. In addition, ensuring children's safety and decreasing risk factors are priorities for clinical attention.

Clinicians assess family dynamics and identify variables that contribute to an emotional or physical climate in which child abuse (especially sexual abuse) can emerge. These family variables are then addressed with the long-term goals of safety and prevention of future abuse. In order to accomplish these tasks, clinicians must often take directive and educational approaches in order to reshape parental responses and thus to ensure more functional and nurturing environments.

In particular, when a child is sexually abused, each member of the family is affected and each person must be included in treatment. In order to maximize lowering family resistance to treatment that is often mandated, a variety of approaches can be utilized. In addition, because young children are involved in treatment, it is helpful to include family play therapy techniques to increase children's participation and to elicit dynamic energy.

As I have noted throughout this book, art, play, and sand therapy are all viable approaches in the treatment of children and adults. These modes of therapy engage unconscious processes through symbols, metaphors, or images, and they require little or no verbalization or explanation to outsiders. As a result, individuals are free to engage in kinetic, sensory, physical, and emotional experiences that have the potential to educate, offer insight, inspire, and cause feelings of well-being. In particular, family play therapy increases opportunities for revealing underlying dynamics, enhancing interactions, relieving tension, and highlighting and pursuing relevant concerns. Family members also often report that it's good to laugh together and have pleasant rather than stressful experiences together.

Family therapy with families in which child sexual abuse occurs includes identification of underlying issues and concerns; trauma-focused work; and eventual restoration of safe and appropriate familial roles, boundaries, and positive interactions. Traditionally, as family members improve their individual functioning, professional team members will taper off or reduce their services. In addition, incestuous child sexual abuse tends to occur in multiproblem families, so a range of therapeutic issues are often identified and addressed by a host of appropriate agencies.

As noted in Chapter Five, the research is supportive of CBT and TF-CBT programs with families, which provide coping skills training, gradual exposure, and behavior management skills. In CBT approaches, providing psychoeducational information about child sexuality and prevention strategies is of paramount importance. In addition, parent–child dyadic therapy has received empirical support and can be pivotal in enhancing conflictual or nonsupportive parent–child relationships. Once again, I encourage clinicians to think about an integrated approach in treating families where child maltreatment (especially sexual abuse) occurs.

7

Special Issues

Posttraumatic Play, Trauma-Focused Play Therapy (TF-PT) and Problems of Dissociation[1]

POSTTRAUMATIC PLAY

"Posttraumatic play" is a unique type of play with specific characteristics: It tends to be literal, repetitive, highly structured, self-absorbed, and joyless (Terr, 1983). As the term "posttraumatic" indicates, such play is often initiated by children who experience something traumatic that is not resolved in other ways (e.g., through parental reassurance, or through withdrawal from the stressor or event and achievement of safety). These children often become engrossed in posttraumatic play activity to the extent that they disregard those around them, experience dissociative episodes, remain unengaged in interpersonal exchanges, and generate or express little visible affect. Clinical observation, documentation, facilitation, and even initiation (through selection of toys or encouragement) of such play by therapists is called "Trauma-Focused Play Therapy." Trauma-

---

[1] Some of the material on posttraumatic play in this chapter was adapted from an article that appeared in the *Association for Play Therapy Newsletter* (1998). Since its initial publication, I have updated and revised this material and now use different case examples. In addition, some of the material on processing dissociation was originally presented in Gil's videotape *Play Therapy for Severe Psychological Trauma: The Theory and Practice of Play Therapy with Trauma* (1998).

focused play therapy (TF-PT) can be initiated or stimulated by clinicians in order to elicit posttraumatic play which can be a child's natural mechanism for gradual exposure to a traumatic incident.

The steps for TF-PT include:

1. Select toys purposefully to represent trauma aspects and to allow child to use them as literal symbols of trauma, making them visible (in a prominent location) in the room.
2. Allow children to approach and engage with selected toys naturally.
3. If children avoid these toys for more than three sessions, direct their attention to the toys and encourage them to play with them.
4. Observe and document thematic material with special attention to sequence and outcome of play.
5. Observe and document repetition of play.
6. Provide verbal narrative during the child's play, providing behavioral descriptions but not interpretations or suggestions.
7. If child is already providing a verbal narrative, encourage the child to expand on the information by asking open-ended questions.
8. Inquire into the play and invite some verbal communication of thoughts, emotions, and behaviors in the play (for example, "How does the bear feel when his mom leaves him alone?" vs. "Why does the bear feel sad?").
9. Observe the evolution in play outcomes: If children introduce healthy adaptive elements, note those; if children get stuck in repetitive play with no change in outcome, introduce the concept of options by stating, for example, "I wonder what the bear wishes might happen right now."
10. Do *not* state solutions for children. Allow them to arrive at those solutions on their own. You can provide two or three possibilities but no specific option.
11. Encourage dynamic movement of some type, either by encouraging movement of toys, giving voices to toys, or asking children to move about the room.
12. When children engage in repetitive play, articulate or listen to narratives of their play, make note when they discharge affect, change the sequence of play to include more adaptive outcomes, and experience a sense of mastery. As a result, they may begin to develop feelings of well-being and restoration of power.
13. Once children have processed their trauma using play therapy, they may be more receptive to psychoeducational information, including group therapy.

Some clinicians place a high priority on accessing posttraumatic play and encourage children to use such play to reap its potential benefits in processing and managing the trauma memory. Other clinicians take a more structured approach to helping children resolve traumatic material and subsequent symptom formation by utilizing (TF-CBT) (see Chapter Five). Still others seek to combine directive and nondirective approaches in order to be of the most help to young traumatized children (Shelby & Felix, 2005). This third approach is the one promoted in this text and illustrated in the cases described below and in later chapters. A discussion of the characteristics and types of posttraumatic play, as well as of my clinical stance toward it and possible specific interventions, is interspersed with the presentation below of Margie's case.

Case Illustration: Margie

Margie was 9 years old when I first met her. She was the only child of a European American couple with severe, chronic alcoholism. After reading about the parents' history, I was shocked that Margie had "fallen through the cracks" and had never been reported to the authorities. She had spent much of her time unsupervised and taking care of herself. When her parents were home and not binge-drinking, Margie literally took care of her parents—cooking for them, taking their clothes off so that they were comfortable sleeping, and helping them to shower.

Margie was referred to me shortly after she had been operated on for appendicitis. She had developed a high fever and somehow got herself to a neighbor's house, where an ambulance was called for her. Margie then had emergency surgery, and her parents could not be located for 6 days after her operation. Needless to say, CPS investigators were called; an emergency petition requested the court to grant immediate custody of Margie to the state; and a warrant for child neglect and child endangerment was issued for Margie's parents. Margie's foster parents reported that she was very quiet, withdrawn, and reluctant to join in family activities. They also stated that she stayed by herself and did not appear comfortable with either adults or children. Margie's foster mother, Mrs. Zion, further commented that Margie appeared extremely skittish about calling attention to herself or asking for anything.

Margie seemed to lack spontaneity or curiosity in our first session. I showed her around the room, trying to spark her interest in any of my toys or play activities. She was not receptive to questions, and I quickly learned that she preferred to sit and look down, with her hair covering her face. She didn't seem particularly uncomfortable being quiet; instead, it was as if she was comfortable letting time pass. I gave her some very soft and malleable plasticine, and she proceeded to squeeze it and mold it, making no particular shape. I did parallel play in our first few sessions, and I was struck by how disengaged she seemed and how her energy seemed so effortlessly contained. She remained unmoved by my invitations to play with toys or art materials. I also asked her to participate in a number of standard assessment activities (building sand worlds; constructing a play genogram; playing the Talking, Feeling, Doing Game), and she politely refused. By the third or fourth session, I had talked to Margie's social worker and had obtained more information about her past.

Margie's parents had severe alcoholism by their own admission, and they had told the investigators that they routinely spent 6–10 days at a time away from the house. They admitted that Margie was often their caretaker, and they seemed genuinely repentant about their behavior. Their resolve to reunify with their daughter was apparent in their willingness to follow each and every directive imposed by the court. It was clear that Margie was quite closely bonded to her parents, as they were to her.

Because I was aware of the circumstances of Margie's hospitalization (i.e., she was home alone, spiked a fever, and had to seek help from neighbors), I made the decision to buy a Playmobil hospital set with an operating room, a recovery room, and an ambulance and stretcher. I hoped that making these toys available would decrease Margie's defenses sufficiently for her to make use of them to begin processing her trauma. As Schaefer (1994) states,

> After a passive helpless experience of trauma, children have a compelling need to actively rework the dramatic elements of the trauma in their play. Adults like to talk out their stressful experiences, while young children are prone to play out these experiences. Coping strategies that confront rather than avoid the event seem to be most effective in resolving trauma symptoms. (p. 301)

I put the boxes of hospital toys in the front of my office, so that when Margie came to her fourth appointment, she saw the unopened boxes with the pictures on the front. Before I knew it, she had asked me to open the boxes, and together we took all the little pieces out of their small plastic bags. By the following session, the toys were available for her to use. Thus began her posttraumatic play, which was as purposeful and structured as could be.

Margie set up the Playmobil hospital toys on a small wooden table. After the second time she did this, it seemed to me that she was actually placing them in approximately the same locations on the table. By the fourth time I had witnessed her play, I was fascinated with the precision and sharpness of her placement of the toys. I felt as if I were watching a movie director who was setting up a scene in exactly the same way, so that no one could detect the discontinuity from one "take" of the scene to the next. The play evolved in the following way:

Margie would begin by setting the Playmobil toys down meticulously and precisely, so that the sequence went from right to left. First came the operating room, then the recovery room—both replete with specific furniture and fixtures duplicating medical scenarios to a T. Margie would set everything down and then push her body into a very cushy couch. She would sit there for a few minutes holding a little girl doll in her hands (she had many choices, but always picked the same small female doll). She would look at the doll and seem to go into a trance for about 1 minute. After this period of sitting and holding the doll, she would grab the ambulance, remove the toy men she had previously affixed to the stretcher, and take them out of the ambulance. She would then place the little girl on the stretcher, have the toy men carry her back to the ambulance, and have the ambulance take off. She would do this by lifting the ambulance—sometimes while making a soft siren sound, at other times while making an engine sound, and at still other times while making no sounds at all. The ambulance would then be parked on the end of the table, and Margie would remove the men carrying the girl on the stretcher and have them walk to the operating room. Once there, she would place the little girl figure on the operating table, and the ambulance assistants would take the stretcher and return to the ambulance. After the small girl doll was placed on the operating table, Margie would once again stare into space for about a minute and then resume play. She would bring the stretcher back to take the little girl to the recovery room. Once there, a nurse would appear with food for the girl; flowers would be placed in a vase; and a nurse would come in and out of the room. Margie would then again stare into space, and finally she would sit back on the couch, looking at the scene she had created. In this play, the little girl always stayed in the recovery room. Amazingly, Margie was able to confine her play to a 50-minute hour with remarkable precision. After she sat back and looked at her scenario, it was time for her to leave.

The first three times Margie repeated this play sequence, I was intrigued. She seemed so absorbed and intense, as if her internal experience was in direct contrast to her constricted appearance. As Ekstein (1966) asserts, traumatized children often make their experiences small (through miniatures) and take active control in the play, and a piecemeal assimilation occurs during repetition of structured sequences that appear rigid. This type of play is therefore a child's natural method of gradual exposure.

During the fourth and fifth sessions, I made several comments to Margie during the play—describing exactly what I was seeing, and being careful not to include my interpretations. I might say, for example, "The little girl is on the stretcher and the ambulance is taking her somewhere," or "The little girl is in an operating room," or "The nurse is bringing some food to the little girl." Whenever I made such a comment, Margie would stop her play, back up onto the couch, and begin the play again. She would not make eye contact with me; she simply retraced her steps and began anew, in a very matter-of-fact manner. After these sessions, it was clear that Margie would not tolerate anything that she perceived as inter-ference in her play, and I made the decision simply to allow her to engage in this compelling play without any demands on my part. At the same time, I decided to videotape these sessions, in order to better understand and document their progression.

I videotaped six consecutive sessions, carefully observing this child's process as well as the sequential, repetitive play. I trusted that there was something important in what she was doing, and I patiently waited for changes in the play. Not only did no changes occur; the exactitude of her play was unforgettable. I checked regularly with her foster mother, Mrs. Zion, to see how Margie was doing throughout the week. Mrs. Zion reported that things had neither improved nor worsened, but she also mentioned an important fact: The last few times when Margie had gone home after therapy, she'd held her side and said that the scar from her appendectomy hurt her. The foster mother noted that the pain would usually subside after a while, but Margie had recently reported feeling nauseated after therapy as well.

The foster mother's descriptions of Margie led me to realize that the posttraumatic play was probably not providing Margie with the neces-sary buffering available through the use of symbols (i.e., a safe distance). Instead of utilizing the play to expose herself gradually to the feared event (or memory of that event), Margie appeared to be having the actual physical and emotional experience of the event. This inability to view or experience the play in an "as if" fashion is typical in "revivification"—the reliving of traumatic events instead of processing a memory and achiev-ing a sense of controlled recall. Revivification can actually become re-traumatizing, in that children are not able to access reparative elements that have the capacity of emerging when the play serves its ultimate pur-pose: mastery.

Characteristics and Potential Benefits of Posttraumatic Play

As mentioned earlier, posttraumatic play is a stylized form of play with several unique characteristics: It is repetitive, literal, and highly struc-tured. Children who utilize posttraumatic play often become so en-grossed with the play that their energy appears constricted, and some of the more common features of play (such as spontaneity, laughter, pretend, and role playing) simply don't appear. In generic play, children often develop themes that are resolved (sublimated) in the natural evolutionary course of the play (e.g., a child makes a scary monster out of clay and then massages the mass, eventually rolling it out into a pancake!). In some instances of posttraumatic play, difficult emotions may persist because the play fails to relieve anxiety or release energy through expression. Instead, the child's play is limited and seems to exclude others, including the therapist.

Although several mental health professionals have documented children's reactions to trauma (Levy, 1982; Schaefer, 1994), Terr's (1983, 1990) research on aftereffects of natural traumas experienced by children may have contributed the most to our understanding of children's posttraumatic play behavior. Terr was able to pursue her interest in posttraumatic play by doing a longitudinal study of a group of elementary school children (now adults) who were kidnapped and buried in a school bus in Chowchilla, California (Terr, 1990). She has specified that posttraumatic play is "different, special, a definable variant of ordinary child's play" (1990, p. 238). She goes on to observe that

> play does not stop easily when it is traumatically inspired. And it may not change much over time. As opposed to ordinary child's play, post-traumatic play is obsessively repeated. It is grim. Furthermore, it requires a certain set of conditions in order to proceed, a certain place, a certain assortment of dolls, certain playmates, or a certain routine. It may go on for years. It repeats parts of the trauma. It occasionally includes a defense or two or a feeble attempt at a happy ending, but post-traumatic play is able to do very little to relieve anxiety. It can be dangerous, too. The problem is [that] post-traumatic play may create more terror than was consciously there when the game started. And if it does dissipate some terror, this monotonous play does it so slowly that it might take more than a lifetime before the play would completely dissipate all the anxiety stirred-up by the trauma. (1990, p. 239)

My own experience with posttraumatic play has confirmed that such play can be both liberating and dangerous. However, I have developed a much more optimistic view of its potential benefits within the context of treatment than the quotation from Terr above might suggest. I regard posttraumatic play as a natural form of self-imposed "gradual exposure" (the CBT technique of attempting to desensitize a person to a feared stimulus through incremental contact with or approach to the stimulus, in order to allow for greater tolerance of affect). The intent of posttraumatic play appears to be mastery and control through repetition (Marvasti, 1993). By utilizing this distinctive type of play, children first externalize the feared or overwhelming event that they may be otherwise avoiding by not thinking or speaking about it (in other words, by suppressing the material and not discussing it with others). Interestingly, while they may make a conscious decision to avoid direct confrontation of traumatic material, they seem compelled to replay the suppressed events by utilizing symbols (toys) that may provide the necessary safe distance so that the material can be approached. Although the posttraumatic play is a quite literal reenactment of the children's actual experience, the children may be able to access the safety provided by symbolic play (in Margie's case, the doll was being operated on, not Margie herself). Children's ability to externalize and narrate their stories through action can allow for gradual integration of feared affect or cognitions. Paradoxically, as children recreate and conclude the play sequence while maintaining a sense of safety and control (i.e., control over how long the play lasts, who says and does what, what does and does not happen), the children may experience a sense of restoration. They are exposed to frightening memories, but the actual events are not happening to them as they construct or dismantle the scene of the trauma. Nader and Pynoos (1991) found that "children's traumatic play may either provoke anxiety or provide relief for a child, perhaps related to the degree of perceived control over outcome, to the degree a satisfactory ending is achieved; to the degree that there is freedom to express the prohibited affect (e.g., revenge), or to the degree a cognitive reworking is facilitated.

Even though the intent of posttraumatic play is mastery, such play also has inherent dangers: If it fails to accomplish its intended goal, traumatized children can actually become retraumatized through the play, experiencing more intense feelings of vulnerability and increased helplessness. This seems to occur when the required emotional distance usually afforded through the use of symbols is not achieved. As Terr (1990) has noted, posttraumatic play can continue for a long time, and it is the uninterrupted (unprotected) type of this play that seems to have problematic implications. I believe that the best outcomes occur when children produce posttraumatic play in a therapy setting, in the presence of a trained clinician who can document the movement of the play, obtain collateral information from caretakers, and initiate interventions as needed (to forestall dangerous impact).

When one is observing posttraumatic play in children, it is necessary to first distinguish between the type of such play that helps address and resolve traumatic material, and the type that hinders, retraumatizes, or elicits greater feelings of vulnerability and helplessness. For purposes of differentiation, I have termed the former type of posttraumatic play "dynamic" and the latter type "stagnant." This distinction allows for more specific discussion of the features or variables of posttraumatic play; more importantly, it can suggest clinical techniques for recognizing and promoting the dynamic type of play and reducing the risks inherent in the stagnant type.

Dynamic versus Stagnant Posttraumatic Play

Differences between the Two Types of Play

Distinguishing dynamic from stagnant posttraumatic play requires careful documentation and focused concentration, since very subtle differences can emerge, signaling that the play may be serving a more reparative or therapeutically or useful purpose. For example, I have found that something as subtle as the location in which the play occurs may denote less rigidity in the play (a feature I associate with dynamic play). Children may also make outcome changes, such as the presence of other objects where none existed before. In order to document miniscule changes, clinicians must truly attune themselves to the play. This need to attend to detail is what initially caused me to videotape posttraumatic play.

Dynamic posttraumatic play has numerous qualitative differences from stagnant play. Over time, children release a broader range of affect; they are physically more fluid and less constricted; they interact with the play and with the therapist in more uninhibited and interactive fashion; the play, although having literal qualities, encompasses departures from rigidity (as noted above) and/or utilizes aspects of pretend play; and finally, children appear emotionally relieved (or fatigued) after engaging in this type of play, rather than tense or shut down. Stagnant posttraumatic play, as its name implies, remains rigid, constricted, serious, and without fluctuations in outcome. Table 7.1 lists variables that can be assessed to determine the type of posttraumatic play a child utilizes and to direct clinical interventions.

Outcomes of Dynamic versus Stagnant Play

As I have emphasized throughout this discussion, posttraumatic play can be thought of as a form of gradual exposure by which children attempt to face traumatic memories and associated affect. Through generic or dynamic posttraumatic play, children contain and manage the memories symbolically by making them concrete (through the use of objects) and then manipulating or changing elements of the play, often producing an increased sense of mastery and control. Children who give themselves this protective cushion can feel their feelings gradually, because they have the control to identify with the objects in the story as much or as little as they can at any given time.

When children change elements in the play, they take an active role on their own behalf and in their own interests; in other words, they go from victims to active change agents. When children nurture, protect, or value their projected selves, they engage in attempts at restoration. When hurtful objects are held accountable, punished, or confined, children are

TABLE 7.1. Differences between Dynamic and Stagnant Posttraumatic Play

Dynamic posttraumatic play	Stagnant posttraumatic play
Affect becomes available	Affect remains constricted
Physical fluidity becomes evident	Physical constriction remains
Interactions with play becomes varied	Interactions with play remain limited
Interactions with clinician become varied	Interactions with clinician remain limited
Play changes, or new elements are added	Play stays precisely the same
Play occurs in different locations	Play is conducted in same spot
Play includes new objects	Play is limited to specific objects
Themes differ or expand	Themes remain constant
Outcomes differ, and healthier, more adaptive responses emerge	Outcomes remain fixed and nonadaptive
Rigidity of play loosens over time	Play remains rigid
After-play behavior indicates release or fatigue	After-play behavior indicates constriction/tension
Out-of-session symptoms may remain unchanged or peak at first, but then decrease	Out-of-session symptoms are unchanged or increase

being restored and fortified. Piaget (1951), in discussing the healing properties of play discusses two types of play behaviors that are noteworthy: "compensatory" and "liquidating." He defines compensatory play behaviors as those that transform a negative emotional experience to make it more pleasing, and liquidating play behaviors as those that allow the emergence and release of strong emotions. I believe that dynamic posttraumatic play has both compensatory and liquidating qualifies. Following this type of posttraumatic play, the more typical opportunities provided by developmental play allow children to compensate for real disappointments or losses.

Conversely, when posttraumatic play does not fulfill its potential and stagnates, children can experience more debilitation, because they are reminded of (and transported to) the overwhelming original trauma and their inability to defend themselves against it. Children who initiate posttraumatic play, but cannot find relief or release, can feel more disheartened, more threatened, and less able to restore and regroup (as if they are being literally retraumatized, which they often are). Thus clinicians must monitor this play carefully and be ready to design and implement interventions designed to redirect, shape, or transform the play from stagnant to dynamic. The presence of the play is almost always an indicator of growth and health (the drive toward resolution). The absence of a positive outcome, however, signals danger as well as the need for clinical guidance.

Clinical Interventions in Posttraumatic Play

When to Intervene

The timing of clinical interventions in posttraumatic play is one of the most pivotal elements in an effective outcome (integration of traumatic material and restoration of preabuse functioning). However, this decision must be made on a case-by-case basis, and there are no rigid or absolute guidelines for it. Intervening too quickly may interfere with the play's inherent capacity to produce positive results; waiting too long may cause the child further revictimization, which (as noted earlier) can reinforce feelings of helplessness and vulnerability. Rubin (1978/1984) notes the use of clinical patience when working with traumatized children (in her case, utilizing art therapy) in order to allow a "working-through" process that she describes as accomplished "through repetitive confrontations with the feared idea, through drawing or playing out a loaded theme, often with a limited amount of modification. While this process may seem like a 'stuck' one to the therapist, it is a necessary one for the child, who may be going through something analogous to a 'desensitization' process, gradually becoming more and more comfortable with previously uncomfortable ideas and feelings" (p. 86).

I have found it useful to document a child's play for a minimum of 6–8 sessions, and then allow another 8–10 sessions to watch for slight variations and to check with caretakers about the child's out-of-session behavior. I then try to determine whether the play has become stagnant, or might still have the potential to be reparative. If I determine that the posttraumatic play is indeed stagnant and potentially damaging to the child, I plan a series of interventions designed to provoke some changes in the play. On occasion I have begun interventions without waiting this long, but the time frame described above serves as a very general basis for my decision making. Needless to say, this particular mode of treatment with traumatized children does not lend itself to rigid, externally imposed schedules.

How to Intervene

There is no one single intervention that will be effective across the board. Instead, I rely on a continuum of interventions, ranging from low-challenge to high-challenge. These clinical interventions are likely to be considered intrusive or disruptive by children who have created a play ritual that by definition is "closed," or exclusive of interaction with others. As children enter this play, they enter the world of traumatic memories, which most likely cannot be initially understood, verbalized, or integrated into larger experiences. It is repetitive because it represents a focal point of children's preoccupation and concern.

Examples of low-challenge/low-intrusion interventions include asking a child to make physical movements (e.g., moving the arms or oxygenating the body) or doing a verbal narration of the child's play (descriptive, not interpretive). High-challenge/high-intrusion interventions include directing the child to one segment of the play (therefore disrupting its sequential rigidity), or videotaping the child's play so it can be viewed by the therapist and child together.

It is critical to remember that if the play does not help resolve the traumatic concerns, questions, or conflicts, it is likely to become stagnant and lose its reparative potential.

Case Illustration: Margie Revisited

Margie was obviously stuck in literal, compulsive, and repetitive play with little resolution or change. Her play remained nondynamic and rigid, while some of her symptoms remained the same and others were becoming worse outside the session.

Margie was unresponsive to many of my low-challenge interventions. As a matter of fact, she often waited until I had made a comment or asked a question, and then quietly and purposefully returned all items to their original starting place—either beginning the play from scratch, or terminating the session early. She was also indifferent to some of my high-challenge interventions, except for the viewing of her play. As soon as I videotaped[2] her posttraumatic play and she watched the play on the television monitor, she made an immediate and stark change in her behavior. As I pointed to the play on the television screen, she seemed to disengage from the play and interact with me—answering my questions about what was going on, and making spontaneous comments such as "She doesn't like what they're doing to her now." My guess is that for some children, the fact that the play is a kinesthetic experience (i.e., toys

---

[2] If clinicians are not able to videotape sessions, they might consider possible substitutes for videotaping, keeping in mind the goal of creating greater distance for the child. Taking still photos or creating a story board might create the desired effect.

are touched, smelled, felt, and manipulated) does not allow them a *safe enough* distance to process the material. My understanding of this phenomenon is that viewing a videotape of the play accentuates the difference between remembering something that has already happened and experiencing a memory as if it were happening anew. In other words, children must eventually believe that their traumatic experiences are being remembered (from the past), not happening currently. One of the potential benefits of posttraumatic play is the pairing of a frightening memory with the experience of current safety—that is, "I am remembering a bad thing, but nothing bad is happening to me."

For Margie, there were several conflicts inherent in her traumatic memory. She felt guilty for "abandoning" her parents, and on some level she felt responsible for the fact that they had been arrested and were now in a treatment program (which she viewed as incarceration). Margie had also felt abandoned herself when her parents did not visit her in the hospital after her surgery. It's also possible that her years and years of loneliness had had a cumulative effect on her. Moreover, her caretaking role was so strongly defined that Margie was concerned that her parents would not survive without her. These were awesome thoughts and feelings for a small child, who was simply unable to cope with them or with the situation.

I felt fortunate to be able to conduct family therapy when Margie's parents were eventually released from their treatment program (after 1 full year). During this time, Margie remained incredibly loyal to them, and her anxiety about them was somewhat dissipated when she could begin phone contact with them after 6 months. The phone calls seemed to nurture her and restore her sense of calm. At the same time, she was often depressed after the calls—perhaps because she was coming to terms with the fact that her parents were indeed surviving without her, bringing her identity and future role into question. Margie and I proceeded into many other areas in treatment, such as her grief and loss, her exaggerated sense of competence (vs. seeing herself as a child who needed attention and nurturance), putting her parents' needs before hers, and the need for her to develop a more accurate self-image. Her relationship with her parents appeared complex, and I was certain that this child had a range of feelings she would need to express before being able to define her identity as separate from theirs.

We had 3 months' notice that the parents would be available for family therapy, and Margie and I prepared well for that encounter. In addition, I was able to meet with the parents a few times prior to the first family session. Both parents had made substantial progress, motivated by their deep love for Margie. They seemed to understand the gravity of their behavior and its possible effects on their child. They had hit the proverbial "rock bottom," and their transformation seemed fragile but genuine.

When we all met together for the first time, the family members' emotions were overwhelming as they hugged and cried together for a full 15 minutes. Eventually the parents guided Margie to calm down so that they could talk a little, stating that they had "lots to tell her." Margie's mother began by telling her that she was clean and sober and felt "new again, as if I had just been born." She went on to say, "Daddy and I realize now that we have been very, very bad parents to you." When Margie protested, her mother hushed her gently: "You have taken care of us instead of the other way around . . . you haven't been able to be a child, because you've had to be taking care of two drunk parents." I could tell that the harsh words surprised Margie, but her father held her hand and added:

> "Yes, Margie, we've been drunk a lot since you were born. Thank goodness that your grandma was able to take care of you the first 4 years of your life . . . we've always loved you, but we've loved ourselves and our drinking more. That stops now. [The resolve in the father's voice was impressive.] It's not going to be easy . . . we've got to keep sober, and that happens one day at a time. Your mom and I have to find jobs and a place that we can afford. Things will take time, but we know you're in a safe place right now, and that gives us the peace of mind to just start building a little place for us so that we can ask the judge to let you come home."

Margie protested again and cried a little, insisting that she was ready to go home immediately. Both parents reassured her that even though she was ready, they would take more time and would only bring her home when they felt that they were going to be able to "do right" by her.

Bittersweet feelings filled the room, and then Margie announced, "I want to show you a videotape." In all the times we had imagined this first meeting and prepared for how Margie would greet her parents or what they might discuss, Margie had never mentioned wanting to show them the tape. When I put it on, Margie walked up to the screen, used her finger to point to it, and narrated her whole story. She used the remote control to stop and start the tape, and she would comment about her thoughts and feelings at specific junctures. For example, when the stretcher carried the little girl from the ambulance to the emergency room, Margie stated: "Here's when I was the most scared. I didn't know what was going to happen. I kept asking people to find you, but they didn't answer me. My stomach hurt a lot, and I couldn't think good. I was really hot in my face, and I was sweaty. I got worried that you'd get home and I wouldn't be there." The parents held hands, cried, and after the tape viewing held Margie in their arms. "We're so sorry that you were alone . . . We wish we could have been there with you . . . How scary for you . . . You've been through so much . . . We're so sorry." Margie seemed to listen and soak up her parents' words.

Margie made considerable progress in therapy after this, and her foster parents allowed her to be more of a child and less of a caretaker. Because Margie's positive self-image derived from her ability to be responsible and take care of others, she was given a few specific chores so that she could be helpful sometimes. At other times, she was told that she had "children's work" to do, and she was told to go outside and play or do homework.

The parents took approximately 6 months to get jobs and find a small apartment. They continued to attend Alcoholics Anonymous and seemed very committed to their programs. They also attended family therapy sessions as requested and met all other demands of the court. Margie was successfully reunited with her family after being in foster care for almost 2 years. I have seen Margie from time to time throughout the years, and she now e-mails me to tell me how she's doing. Her father was able to maintain his sobriety, but her mother has had a few relapses, and Margie's parents separated a few years back. Margie is determined to become a nurse.

PROBLEMS OF DISSOCIATION

Case Illustration: Cassie

Cassie was a 5-year-old Hispanic child who presented with many of the early symptoms (and detachment) I saw in Margie. Cassie had been sexually abused by her uncle and two other adult males during their production of child pornography. She had been forced to copulate orally with adult males, as well as to "lie still" while adult males copulated orally with her. The abuse had occurred weekly over a 2-month period. The police confiscated photographs that fully substantiated the horror this child had experienced. A truly compelling feature of these photographs was the blank, vacant, and frightened stare in Cassie's eyes.

Cassie was referred for treatment shortly after she was placed in a loving and secure foster home. She appeared to have little reaction to any life events, including her transfer to foster care. She did not ask about her father, who had been her primary caretaker since her mother's death 2 years prior. She did not hold onto toys or blankets. Mostly she wanted to stay in her bed and suck her thumb.

During therapy Cassie was despondent, with very low energy and absolutely no interest in any play materials. I had never seen a child who was so unresponsive to human interactions. She usually sat in a chair or on the floor, staring blankly as time ticked away. She did not respond to any of my overtures, and my giving her space was equally frustrating, because she would separate herself even more.

Finally, I brought a new doll into the playroom, and I told Cassie a story. I brought the doll wrapped in a blanket, and I made a fuss about the fact that she was brand new, that I had just gotten her, and that she had been badly hurt. I whispered to Cassie, "Sometimes bad things happen to little girls. This little one has been hurt very badly, and she feels scared about everything and everybody." I took the doll and made almost exaggerated motions as I made the doll comfortable, placed her in a bed with the brand-new blanket, got the doll a very small teddy bear, and confided to Cassie, "I'm not sure how to make her feel safe. All I can do is keep trying." Looking at Cassie, I placed the doll in her lap, saying, "Maybe you know how to make her feel better." I then added, "I know. Maybe she can go home with you so that she feels better." Cassie blinked her eyes in acknowledgment, and she began to look at the doll, to open and close the doll's eyes with her finger, and eventually to caress the doll's hair. I won't say she hugged the doll, but she definitely carried her out with her as we ended the session.

Slowly but surely, Cassie began to participate with me in the treatment. Each week she would bring her doll, K. C., and would make her Play-Doh food, bathe her, try on new clothes, comb her hair, and take her to visit the doctor. The foster mother confided that Cassie took the doll with her everywhere and seemed to whisper in her ear constantly. The foster mother also told me that Cassie was participating with the other family members more and more, and that they had instinctively learned to talk to Cassie and include Cassie in their activities.

Over the next 2 months, Cassie made great progress. She often asked for things from others; she sought out physical proximity; she slept better; and her appetite increased. She even seemed to tolerate playing with a next-door neighbor. At the same time, there were some disturbing behaviors. She would often sit still, staring blankly; also, her hygiene was very poor, with frequent bedwetting or soiling of her pants during the day.

Eventually two primary processes became clear for therapeutic consideration: (1) Cassie was "spacing out" whenever she felt afraid, lonely, or sad; and (2) she seemed to disregard her genitals, as if they were not there. When I asked her to draw her self-portrait, she drew a head, arms that came out of the head, and ankles and feet at the bottom of the page. It was as if she pretended that her genitals did not exist, because these parts of her body had produced pain and discomfort. Both of these processes were dissociative responses, which often go undiagnosed and untreated in children.

Forms and Functions of Dissociation

The phenomenon of dissociation was first discussed by Pierre Janet (1925). Dissociation is considered an effective coping strategy under some conditions, but can be an impediment to healthy functioning in others; it may occur either episodically or chronically. Dissociative disorders were introduced as a new diagnostic category in DSM-III (American Psychiatric Association, 1980), and DSM-IV-TR currently defines dissociation as "a disruption in the usually integrated functions of consciousness, identity, memory, or perception" (American Psychiatric Association, 2000, p. 519). In addition to describing dissociative disorders per se, DSM-IV-TR includes "dissociative flashback episodes" (American Psychiatric Association, 2000, p. 468) among the possible symptoms of PTSD.

Dissociation occurs along a continuum, the most extreme form being "dissociative identity disorder," or DID (formerly known as "multiple personality disorder"). This condition is the existence within a person of "two or more distinct identities or personality states (each with its own relatively enduring pattern of perceiving, relating to, and thinking about the environment and self)" (American Psychiatric Association, 2000, p. 529). At least two of the identities or personality states recurrently take control of the person's behavior. DID has received a great deal of attention from researchers and clinicians throughout history, but the 1980s and early 1990s saw a proliferation of literature on the subject (Kluft, 1985; Braun & Sachs, 1985; Putnam, 1989; Ross, 1991), and more recent works have focused on childhood dissociation (Shirar, 1996; Silberg, 1996a) and dissociation as an aspect of PTSD in children (Silva, 2004). The research and development of assessment instruments for childhood dissociation is aptly discussed in Peterson's (1996) comprehensive chapter. In addition, Silberg (1996b) describes five domains of treatment for dissociative children: cognitive, affective, physical, interpersonal, and spiritual.

In my experience, unless abuse has been extremely severe and bizarre, clinicians are not likely to encounter a high percentage of children with DID. At the same time, it's important to note that DID is thought to occur in children under the age of 7, so it's important to assess for this carefully—particularly in young children who *have* undergone severe, bizarre, chronic, or sadistic abuse.

Forms of dissociation that occur at the lower end of the continuum (such as the symptoms seen in Cassie) include "depersonalization," in which the customary feeling of one's own reality is replaced by a feeling of being detached or estranged from the self. Many individuals who depersonalize describe a sensation of leaving their bodies and observing themselves from a safer vantage point. This process allows trauma survivors to detach themselves from the overwhelming terror of the moment. Unfortunately, it can also disrupt memory of the event and create an identity crisis. "Psychogenic amnesia" is a marked inability to recall important personal information, generally of a stressful or traumatic nature. "Psychogenic fugue" occurs when the individual takes physical flight and has no recollection of the travel after regaining consciousness.

Dissociative processes, initially protective in nature, can become problematic when individuals dissociate in what they perceive to be an uncontrolled fashion, or when individuals experience disturbances in memory with accompanying feelings of disorientation, helplessness, and terror. Like DID, these less extreme dissociative conditions have been the subjects of significant professional study and discussion since the 1980s (Goodwin, 1985; Pynoos & Eth, 1986; van der Kolk, 1987).

Clients who dissociate may not even be cognizant of their dissociative processes; if they are aware of these, they may believe that they are symptoms of mental illness, and therefore may be unwilling or reluctant to bring up the topic. (Many such clients are surprised to find out that other people have similar experiences, and they report feeling less stigmatized as others share their experiences.) Because of this reluctance to discuss dissociation, I have found it useful to initiate therapeutic dialogues with clients who appear to "space out" (take flight) during therapy sessions; who report problems in "feeling real," staying emotionally present, or remembering recent or past events; or who demonstrate other dissociative symptoms.

Assessing, Discussing, and Intervening in Dissociation

Several assessment instruments can be used with adults to document their familiarity with and use of dissociative mechanisms, and to determine the extent of their use. With children, I may have parents or significant caretakers report their observations of the children's behaviors; obviously, children may be even more reluctant than adults to self-report dissociation. For both children and adults, I take the following steps to facilitate discussion:

1. *Develop a language for the process of "dissociation."* The first step in discussing dissociation is to agree upon a language for it. With children, I may make explicit the behaviors I have just observed—for example, "Cassie, I notice that sometimes you sit leaning on the wall, you stare at the wall in front of you, you suck your thumb, and you seem to go away."

Then I ask, "What do you call it when you do that?" Most people call it "spacing out," although other descriptions include "zoning out," "getting little," "going inside," or "daydreaming." If children cannot acknowledge these behaviors, I may (with their permission) videotape sessions and show them what they may not be able to remember.

2. *Assess typical uses of dissociative responses.* Once a preferred language is established, clients may be able to discuss their use of dissociation. Does it occur at specific times of the day? What's usually going on right before they do it, or right afterward? Typical responses range from boredom, fatigue, and stress to fear, anxiety, and arousal. If children say, "I don't know," you might tell them that they probably know more than they think, and you would like them to pay attention to what they notice next time they do it.

3. *"Normalize" dissociation and describe it as adaptive in some situations.* I explain to children that everybody dissociates (using their language for it), and that some people do it more than others. I tell them that for most people, dissociation is initially a helpful strategy. I then ask children to think about ways that dissociating helps them out. Dissociation should be described as the creative defensive strategy that it is.

4. *Discuss the disadvantages of dissociation.* At the same time, it is important for clients to consider that dissociative responses can have their disadvantages. For example, if someone is driving a car, that would not be a good time to "space out." Likewise, if a child is at school and the teacher is teaching a lesson, dissociating would not be a helpful thing to do. Ask clients if there are times when dissociating becomes problematic, especially if it's used excessively and results in their feeling out of control, helpless, and scared. Talk about times when the clients would rather not dissociate. Review the advantages and disadvantages that have been identified during this discussion.

5. *Obtain a contract for intervening in unhelpful dissociation.* The goal of working with clients who dissociate is to heighten their ability to dissociate at will. Dissociation is disruptive and problematic when it occurs out of a client's perceived control, when it causes depersonalization, or when it interferes with memory. An adult survivor of child abuse who was attending group therapy confided, "I hate it that I miss most of what's said in group. Every week I go determined to 'stay with' the group process, and every week something triggers me and I can't stay present." Having shared her feelings of frustration and despair over not being able to control her dissociative processes, this client readily agreed to work on obtaining more control.

6. *Establish the sequence of dissociative responses.* Everyone who dissociates has a unique way of initiating an episode, although it is usually out of conscious awareness. Focusing a client on the cognitive, affective, sen-

sory, physiological, and behavioral components that precede a dissociative episode is instrumental in tracking the sequence of dissociation. I ask clients to conduct an experiment at their earliest convenience (sometimes this can be done in the therapy hour), in which they "pretend" to dissociate; they should notice what they say to themselves, what their bodies do, and any sensations or feelings they have. Clients have returned with responses ranging from "I focus on a spot on the ceiling," to "I lie down or sit down in a certain way," to "I close my eyes and hold my breath," to "My face feels flushed and my breathing gets shallow." I encourage clients to identify the earliest clue of their dissociation. They are usually surprised to see how early in the process they notice a difference on some level. If they are able to identify the earliest point, that point is labeled the "point of intervention"—that is, the earliest moment when an alternative behavior can occur to interrupt the dissociative response. I point out that clients have more choice at this point than later in the cycle, when momentum is gained.

Interventions vary for each client, and experimentation is encouraged. I find that physical movement and oxygenating the body are effective ways to interrupt the sequence of dissociation. At times, clients find that talking to themselves or speaking to those around them may be effective. As with anything else, practice is helpful—and the more alternative strategies designed and tested, the better. The client who wanted to be more present during group therapy would raise her hand, stand up, and announce that she was in danger of spacing out. She would then ask for the group's help to stay emotionally available.

7. *Explore alternatives to flight: Affect tolerance.* Because dissociation effectively protects an individual from feared affect, affect tolerance and modulation are not achieved. If a client is not able to feel his or her feelings, those feelings remain mysterious and foreboding. I encourage clients to stretch their tolerance for affect by consciously choosing to struggle through their fear an inch at a time. When clients express the precipitating fear associated with the flight response, I ask them to "stand their feeling" for 10, 30 or 50 seconds more. Eventually the time is extended as clients see for themselves that feelings can be tolerated and they will not be consumed or obliterated by them.

Once the triggers that elicit dissociative responses have been identified, clients can work on understanding the origin of these feelings; developing alternative responses to flight urges; appreciating the potential benefits of controlled dissociation; and developing healthy and constructive ways of tolerating, discharging, and managing affect. Dissociation has been an effective internal coping resource for many individuals with histories of trauma. At the same time, when dissociative responses are experienced as spontaneous, disruptive, and problematic, clients can benefit from careful exploration of alternative affective and behavioral responses. The goal with any survivor of trauma is to bring the trauma to conscious awareness and process the material so that the survivor can achieve a sense of empowerment and control. This structured approach is one of the means toward that end. When individuals are able to curtail unwanted dissociative responses, they will have fewer memory gaps and feelings of depersonalization.

If feelings of depersonalization persist, I have found it useful to design interventions that assert feelings of humanity. In particular, when children have told me about not feeling parts of their bodies, or feeling as if they are watching themselves from outside their bodies, I explore creative ways to assist them in feeling the boundaries of their physical and spiritual selves. Some physical strategies include having clients lower and raise their pulse rates; listen to their heartbeats; engage in physical activity and observe their capacity for sweating; take snapshots that can be reviewed and described; look in the mirror and describe the image they see; and so forth. Nonphysical strategies include meditation or prayer; journal writing; drawing, painting, or sculpting; chanting; participating in group activities; and engaging in any other activities that promote a sense of self-expression, improved self-esteem, and affiliation with others.

SUMMARY

Posttraumatic play serves an important function in children's reparative process and has tremendous potential benefits. However, such play can also be dangerous to children if it does not meet its intended goals. Distinguishing between posttraumatic play that is helpful (dynamic) and play that is possibly dangerous (stagnant) will allow clinicians to shape specific behavioral interventions that restore the play's original potential. Careful observation and documentation of posttraumatic play must guide clinical decisions to allow or challenge the play.

There is a link between trauma and dissociation, and it is not uncommon for children to have a range of dissociative problems when they have experienced trauma. Problems of dissociation are challenging when they appear in clinical situations, and must be understood and addressed in order to ensure children's full participation and benefit in therapy. Problems of "spacing out," not "feeling real," or not feeling parts of the body are more common forms of dissociation in children and can be addressed through a variety of directive and nondirective strategies.

PART II

Four Case Illustrations

8

Scotty, the Castle, and the Princess Guard

REFERRAL INFORMATION

Scotty, a 6-year-old African American child, was referred by his department of family services (DFS) social worker when a concern arose about
possible sexual abuse in a prior foster home. The most urgent presenting
problem was that Scotty had developed selective mutism.

PSYCHOSOCIAL HISTORY

Scotty had experienced a great deal of abuse and upheaval in his first
few years of life. His records documented a history of sexual abuse, inconsistent care, and multiple caretakers. He was initially placed in foster care at the age of 8 months because of parental neglect due to drug
addiction. A neighbor mercifully called the police when she heard a
loud altercation in the next apartment and saw the adults leave without
their infant, who cried for about 20 minutes before falling asleep. The
police found Scotty unattended, malnourished, and lying on the floor.
He was placed with his maternal grandmother, who had previously
been unaware of his existence. She was apparently a frail, sickly woman
who cared for Scotty the first 3 years of his life until she died suddenly
in a car accident. He was then placed with another relative (a young

aunt with two children), and the case was closed with DFS. However, when Scotty's aunt divorced, she sent Scotty to live with more distant relatives. During this shuffling around, Scotty once again came to the attention of DFS when his day care provider called the agency after noticing blood in Scotty's underwear. Due to the extended family's inability to secure a stable or safe placement, he was transferred to a pre-adoption foster home in which there were four other male children, two of whom had been adopted by the family.

After nearly 1 year, this placement was aborted as a result of a sexual abuse allegation. Three of the younger children reported that an older child in placement was sexually abusing them while they tried to sleep. An investigation revealed that the younger children were being terrorized by the older child, who threatened them into compliance with sexual acts (oral sex and masturbation). It was unclear whether Scotty also fell victim to this older child, but his prior history of sexual abuse at the age of 4 (anal intercourse) was documented by both medical evidence and his allegation, although the identity of his abuser was never known. Whether Scotty was abused by this older child (he denied he was) or watched as this boy abused his roommates (which was also unclear, because the other boys claimed that Scotty slept through everything), Scotty had sudden, acute symptoms of PTSD (hypervigilance, etc.) and of dissociation ("spacing out" and extreme forgetfulness).

Scotty was referred to treatment when he was placed in his second foster home. The referring query was for an evaluation to determine whether Scotty had been sexually abused in his first foster placement. In addition, Scotty had stopped talking at home or school, and appeared fearful, anxious, and sad.

ISSUES SUGGESTED BY PRESENTING PROBLEMS (DECODING OF SYMPTOMS)

My understanding of Scotty's presenting problems was developed in the context of the facts presented to me, as well as what I could imagine had been a more global environment of inconsistency, danger, injury, and lack of gentle attention and nurturing. He had been left alone by his drug-addicted parents; he had been shuffled from one relative to another in his earliest years; he had experienced one documented incident of acute sexual abuse; and he had been exposed to sexual abuse in his first foster home. It was no wonder he didn't want to speak. He had been terrorized and probably had very few expectations of rewarding experiences from the world. He was frozen in his little body, expecting that adults would hurt him or ignore him. His world of silence likely provided a sanctuary in which he could be safe and retreat into fantasy. My first and most critical challenge was showing this child that not all people would hurt him. What a monumental and important task to achieve!

RISK TO SELF AND OTHERS

Sexually abused children, especially males, may develop aggressive behaviors toward others. This was not the case with Scotty. Scotty had no visible signs of aggression; instead, he was consumed with dread, since the world had shown itself to be consistently dangerous.

Scotty had also not developed self-harming behaviors, as other injured children might do. He did not hit, bite, or otherwise hurt himself physically. Therefore, the risk he posed to either himself or others appeared low. His selective mutism obviously suggested that he was in great emotional distress; however, I viewed this behavior as the child's attempt to help himself, and I knew that Scotty might be interested in speaking again if the environment could be made safe. I kept thinking that he would first have to have someone to talk with, and, later, something to ask for or something to say.

SYSTEMIC ISSUES

Scotty's current physical environment seemed more than adequate. He had been placed in another preadoption foster home with a single African American mother who seemed kind and interested. When she brought Scotty to sessions, she spoke to him quietly, held his limp hand, and constantly touched his head and face. She seemed like a lovely mother bird, trying to wrap her wings around the child. Scotty often elicited this response from adults, because he was small and frail-looking, with huge, sad eyes that often looked to the floor.

There were obvious systemic issues in Scotty's past. He had experienced multiple settings; multiple foster care workers; and many apparently uninterested, busy, or reluctant caretakers. He'd probably never developed a sense that he belonged anywhere or to anyone, and the opportunity for him to develop a secure attachment had not occurred, except perhaps with his grandmother in the first 3 years of his life (her death had probably been a significant loss for Scotty). The most critical systemic goal was permanent placement, with the opportunity for a stable, safe, and loving home.

PARENTAL COACHING

During the course of an evaluation, it is important to stay actively involved with a parent or other primary caretaker, in order to ascertain the impact of the treatment sessions; to learn about changes in the child's immediate environment; and to exchange information about how the parent or caretaker can promote therapy work and how the therapist can promote parental messages within treatment. In order to achieve these purposes, coaching sessions with parents/caretakers are held. In my experience, parents usually need direction about how much or little to say to children about their past abuse, how to shape desirable behaviors, how to encourage them, and how to speak with them.

Scotty's foster mother, Darlene, was my best ally. She was a ferocious protector—"just what the doctor ordered" to counteract Scotty's previous experiences. She and I talked frequently, and my plan was to incorporate her into the therapy whenever I could. Without breaking confidentiality, I explained to her that Scotty was working on boundary issues, dealing with his fear and anxiety, and processing difficult emotional material. I always took pictures of Scotty's work, and sometimes he took his creations home. Darlene surmised the meaning of the work without my needing to explain much. She comforted Scotty, read to him, and created an environment in which he could develop a sense of safety. She kept his room clean and tidy; she didn't overwhelm him with toys; she constructed a routine for bedtime and dinner; and she drove him to and from school. He eventually responded to her consistent care and attention.

The only coaching I felt necessary was to help Darlene understand that Scotty would not necessarily find all this positive attention comfortable. In fact, I asked her to "tone down" her positive commentary to him for the time being. She understood immediately, and soon proudly announced she had only told him twice in a week how handsome and smart he was. Of course, eventually this positive praise could be given without concern, but initially Scotty cringed when personal comments were made by others.

During the last few sessions, I mentioned to Scotty that he could invite Darlene into the room and show her around. He did so with great pride, showing her the sand trays he had used, the art materials, and other objects in the room. Darlene listened and showed interest.

Darlene and I spoke often during the course of treatment, and we met once a month in an individual session. With other parents or caretakers, more direct work will be necessary to ensure therapy's progress. Indeed, sometimes parents must attend therapy sessions themselves, because the assessment has indicated that a disruption in the parent–child relationship is contributing to the child's inability to adapt to the environment or to control problem behaviors.

As a trained family therapist, I think systemically and invite family members to participate in a variety of talk therapy sessions as well as expressive therapy sessions (see Chapter Six). I don't have any strict rules that apply in all cases, but I remain in constant communication with family members both in and out of therapy sessions.

TREATMENT PLAN

Based on the history that was provided to me, my understanding of how Scotty's presenting problems (or symptoms) had emerged in the context of his history, his current low level of risk to self or others, and the critical overall systemic goal, my plan was to proceed with a nondirective, low-stress, low-demand therapy situation. I would be patient and present. I would not exhibit too many overt signs of affection or make too many personal remarks that might make Scotty feel too visible and thus less safe. I would take the pressure about talking to me off him by telling him that we could be together in silence. I would meet with Scotty individually at first, and if Darlene continued to exhibit an interest in adopting him, I would invite her for conjoint sessions.

TREATMENT GOALS

My first goal was to conduct a play-based extended developmental assessment (see Chapter Two), utilizing a nondirective approach. My second goal was to decrease Scotty's fear and anxiety. I would enlist Darlene's help in creating a safe external environment.

INDICATORS OF TREATMENT PROGRESS

Progress toward the first goal would be measured by growth in my knowledge of Scotty's functioning, including physical functioning, patterns of interaction, affective expression, play themes, behaviors in and out of therapy, self-reports, and reports from caretakers.

Progress toward the second goal would be measured by Scotty's use of language; his abilities to volunteer information, to ask for help, to sleep through the night, and to take certain risks; his increased physical mobility; his expanded affective capacity; and his ability to negotiate new situations with greater confidence and less resistance.

TIME FRAME

Luckily, DFS personnel had told me that they would pay for whatever therapy I felt Scotty needed, and that there were no time restrictions. I believed that it would take a good 3 months to complete an assessment with Scotty (12 sessions), and then another 6–9 months to provide both individual and family treatment.

PLAY TECHNIQUES

As usual, the play therapy office was stocked with a full array of toys, games, sand trays, and art supplies. I made sure that there were African American dolls, including grandparents (these were important because Scotty's earliest home had been with his grandmother). I also had large and small male and female African American dolls (the male dolls were especially important, given the allegation of sexual abuse by a male teenager in the last foster home and the presence of three other boys). In addition, I had an African American male baby doll, bathtub, crib, and baby bottles, as well as multiple play houses so that Scotty could distinguish between his old house and his new house. Finally, because Scotty had experienced malnutrition, I made sure that play food, bowls, and saucers were available.

THERAPY SESSIONS

I came out to greet Scotty when he arrived for the first session. He sat in a large chair, looking scared and small. I bent down (my knees were still working then) and spoke quietly: "Hi, Scotty, my name is Dr. Gil." He looked down as his foster mother said, "This is the doctor I told you about, Scotty. She's going to help you." I looked at Scotty again, wondering how on earth I could make him feel safer. "I'm not a regular doctor. I won't look in your ears and throat, and I won't give you shots." I took a deep breath. "I have lots of toys in my office, and we'll just play. I hear you don't talk right now, and I want you to know that's just fine with me. We don't have to talk. We can be quiet when we play." I stood up and asked the foster mom to come with us. Darlene took his hand and led him down the hallway, reassuring him: "See, Scotty, she's real nice, and she wants to get to know you, and she wants to help you feel better." I wondered if Scotty could understand the concept that he could feel better or that someone might want to help him. He followed quietly without protesting. He had given up protesting many years back and found it best to be compliant. ("Someday I'm going to hope he acts out big-time," I said to myself, hoping for this child to experience childhood someday.)

In the first and subsequent therapy sessions, I showed Scotty around the play therapy room, often picking up toys and demonstrating their use. He was reserved and hesitant, remaining unresponsive to my efforts to have him hold, manipulate, or select toys that he liked. Indeed, he needed many reassurances before he would even look around or touch things. During these early sessions, Scotty also held his breath quite a bit, stood motionless, and seemed to constrict his muscles. There were periods when he stared away and rocked in place. He was hypervigilant and sensitive to noises outside the room. His startle response seemed delayed (he would flinch a few seconds after noises occurred). It took him at least six sessions to exhibit physical relaxation.

In these initial sessions, I was racking my brain for how to make Scotty feel as comfortable as possible. I gave him lots of space: I pushed my chair into a corner of the room, avoided eye contact, and hummed as I played with various toys. Using my peripheral vision, I could see that Scotty often stole glances around the room, and he held a ball tightly in his right hand. Anxious children can become more anxious during these initial sessions if they don't know how long the sessions will last, or when they will be able to leave. I set a timer for Scotty and told him that when the marker reached zero, the bell would ring and it would be time to go; Scotty watched the timer closely. I also reassured him that his foster mom, Darlene, was in the waiting room, and that he could check to make sure that she was there as often as he wanted. Of course, Scotty never took the initiative to go check on Darlene.

I also told Scotty that the door could stay open or closed (he preferred it to stay a little open, although he signaled this with only the slightest blink of the eyes), and I made sure that he knew where the bathroom and drinking water were. Amazingly, he stayed the entire 50 minutes of each session and didn't bolt out when the bell rang.

In the fifth session, I decided to reintroduce Scotty to the sand trays. I took off the top of the first sand tray, showed him the fine white sand, and used my hand to pick up and release sand. Scotty looked somewhat attentive; at least, it was the first time he showed any change in expression. He maintained his distance from the tray, however. I then showed him the second sand tray (which was for wet sand), and it had a water container nearby. When I poured some water on the sand, he almost gulped audibly. A little splash of water fell on his hand, and he took his finger and rubbed the drop into his skin. ("One day I'm going to take out the finger paints and get him good and immersed in paints," I thought. I wondered how long I would have to wait for that.)

I told Scotty that he was welcome to use the sand trays if and when he wanted, and he watched carefully as I again took sand in my hand, let it run through my fingers, and showed him the blue color on the bottom of the box. I mentioned to him that this blue could be water, sky, or anything else. I put a little fish in a blue circle. "See, there's a little fish in the water. I wonder how that little fish feels being there alone in the water." Scotty looked up at me. I looked back and put another fish in. "There, now he has a friend." (I was interested in my being directive at this point, given that I am usually more patient and I will wait until a child initiates play. However, I perceived something so powerful about Scotty's sense of being alone that I wanted to "tickle his defenses" and try to elicit a response. I remember saying to myself, "You've got to watch your countertransference." I set up a consultation the following day and discussed the countertransferential responses that were creeping in strongly.) Scotty seemed to glance over to the fish and sea shells quite a bit, but he still wasn't picking anything up.

The foster mother told me that prior to our next session (after the "fish and friend" incident), Scotty picked up his coat as if to indicate to her that it was time to leave for therapy. He did this about 5 minutes before it would have been time to leave for the appointment. At this sixth session, Scotty was still withdrawn and fearful, but he put his hand on the sand tray top as if to indicate he wanted me to take the top off. I said to him, "You're putting your hand on the top. Maybe you want to see the sand." I came over and took the top off. This time he put his hand inside the tray. I tried to hold back my intense enthusiasm, and didn't move for fear I'd spook him. I slowly took a chair and pulled it up beside him.

He did sensory play for the most part. He poured sand from one cup to another, and moved sand from one half of the tray to the other, making little piles—a precursor to his later play in the sand. He then picked up a little shell that had been left in the sand, and showed it to me with an expression of wonder. I brought over the container for the shells and said, "Someone left a shell in the sand. This is the jar for the shells." Instead of putting the shell back, Scotty took other shells and started lining them against the four walls of the tray. ("He's reinforcing the boundaries of the tray," I thought to myself. "He's trying to reinforce boundaries to create safety.")

Scotty continued this reinforcement with shells at the next two meetings. He also began to move in a quicker and more relaxed manner around the room, and his selecting and manipulating toys showed me that he was beginning to come out of his shell at last. ("Okay, you're making progress, he's feeling safer," I said to myself.) It was interesting to note that Scotty kept watching the timer throughout these sessions, and when the bell rang, he simply stopped what he was doing and started for the door. I noted his obvious need for clear boundaries, and his adeptness at quick endings and moving on. (Much later in our treatment, he sought to reset the timer on occasion, and began to want to stay longer and longer beyond the bell's ring. Perhaps he was testing the limits of my boundaries, and perhaps he was relaxing his own need to comply rigidly out of fear.)

At about the eighth session, Scotty put his hand on the wet tray. "You want me to open that one," I said. (I always kept the sand tray tops on for this child. His putting his hand on the top was a huge accomplishment.) I complied, and moved this sand tray to the center of the room so he would have ample room to walk around the tray as he worked with it.

The first time Scotty tried to pour water in the tray, he showed palpable anxiety (he held his breath, blinked his eyes rapidly, and made jerky motions). He first put his hand in the container ever so lightly and dripped some drops from his fingers onto the sand. He looked at me immediately, and I wondered if he was expecting me to chastise him. Next he experimented gingerly with pouring a little water into a cup and then into the tray. The act of pouring large amounts of water, which he later did with great abandon, was a slow metaphor for trusting himself and his own controls. Over the next few sessions, he began to pour water more purposefully. He poured just enough to dampen the sand so that he changed its texture. He would then drag his fingers as if lifting the sand with his fingers (reminiscent of turning the earth) and then pat it down completely until it was very flat. When he was through, he would leave the sand flat and would ask me to put the top on by pointing to the lid.

It was during this time that Scotty began to speak outside the therapy sessions, both to his foster mother and to a peer who was befriending him at school. His teacher noted that Scotty seemed more relaxed, went out for recess with the other children, was eating better, and had made a friend. In addition, she said that Scotty would talk to her from time to time but still seemed shy. His treatment team—the foster mother, the teacher, myself, and Scotty's social worker—were very happy with his growth. He still did not speak to me in therapy, but I acknowledged with him that I understood he was now using his voice with his foster mom and his friend. He smiled when I talked to him about this, and I reassured him, "Whenever you want to use your voice in here, I'll be happy to listen to your words just like I listen to your play." He looked away and maintained his control over speaking.

After about four more sessions, Scotty's sand play changed again. He began to push the damp sand aside, creating (blue) circles that resembled water. He then tried to fill these circles with water. He was frustrated by the fact that the water would not "hold," but rather was absorbed into the sand. Eventually, showing great resourcefulness, he brought a piece of plastic to therapy. He made his usual circles and then placed the plastic in the circle. When he poured the water, he found that the water was contained and would not be absorbed by the sand. Finally, he placed a boat in the water. Sure enough, the boat floated, and he offered me a full smile for the first time.

After several sessions of making several circles and filling them with water and floating boats, Scotty turned his attention to the fact that he could "build up" the sand by cupping it together into what appeared to be small mounds. He was fascinated by the fact that wet sand could be molded, and he later discovered on his own that when he put wet sand in a cup and turned the cup over, structures could be placed in the sand. Thus began a particularly interesting form of play, which I viewed as posttraumatic play (see Chapter Seven). This became the primary mode of therapy for Scotty from this moment forward.

POSTTRAUMATIC PLAY

Simply put, posttraumatic play is a repetitive and rigid type of play, initiated by children in an effort to expose themselves to literal aspects of their trauma that cause them despair. I regard it as similar to the CBT technique of gradual exposure: The children expose themselves to difficult information, tolerating more and more affect as they interact with the play, and eventually desensitizing themselves and achieving controlled recall and a subsequent feeling of power and control. I view this as a natural reparative mechanism, because it often produces a critical shift that allows for disengagement from previously overwhelming memories. (See Chapter Seven for a detailed discussion.)

Scotty's posttraumatic play included gradual changes that indicated movement. He first made round mounds (see Figure 8.1). This was followed by his inserting a finger in each mound to make a deep hole (Figure 8.2). Once the mounds with holes had been made at least six times, during six different sessions, he began to insert objects in the holes (Figure 8.3)—filling them up, and often jamming objects so that they created rips along the sides.

During the sessions in which Scotty inserted objects into the holes, his affect became visibly agitated. He seemed very engaged with the process in the sand, often licking his lips, blinking his eyes, and making jerky physical movements. He did not look up during this play, in marked con-

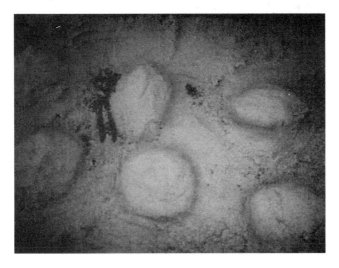

FIGURE 8.1. Scotty's mounds in the sand.

trast to his typical hypervigilance and the way he usually scanned the environment. He grunted and grimaced on occasion.[1]

I was tempted to intervene into Scotty's process by making observations, providing comfort and reassurance, or asking questions. However, I resisted this temptation and decided to respect the process that seemed underway. Because the posttraumatic play seemed dynamic—it evolved naturally and included elements of change—I refrained from what I thought might interfere with his instinctive process.[2] Instead, I sat quietly but remained very emotionally present, witnessing Scotty's self-disclosure and trauma processing. It seemed that each time he reenacted this play in the sand, he was able to tolerate his feelings more and more. The foster

---

[1] My interpretation of Scotty's play may seem obvious to readers: It appeared to me that Scotty was behaviorally reenacting his own anal rape by creating mounds with openings (buttocks and anus); making rips along the sides (his medical records indicated two tears around his anus); and jamming objects inside the openings (his grunts may have reflected grunts he heard during the abuse, or he himself may have expelled grunts as the abuse was forced upon him). His grimacing conveyed pain and despair.

[2] As discussed in Chapter Seven of this text, posttraumatic play can be helpful or retraumatizing for children, depending on many variables. One variable that I believe indicates that the play is dynamic and is serving a positive purpose is whether changes occur during the course of the play. Scotty's play was largely repetitive for several sessions, but it showed visible innovations that signaled his steps toward mastery.

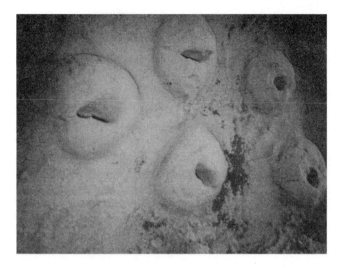

FIGURE 8.2. Holes in the mounds.

mother mentioned during this time that Scotty's nightmares were becoming less frequent and less intense.

Scotty then added other elements to his play. He took the large water container, filled it up, and brought it next to the sand tray. He also brought over a towel. After the play reached its conclusion (making mounds, creat-

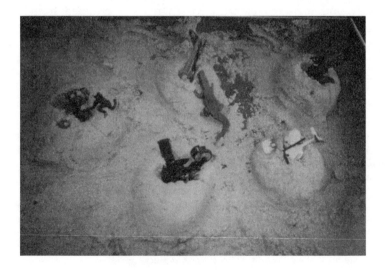

FIGURE 8.3. Objects in the mounds.

ing holes, and inserting objects into the holes), he took the toys out of the sand, dropped them in the container of water, and then dried them with a towel. He also put liquid soap in the container of water. When he took the toys out of the bubbly water, he took them one by one to the towel, and then quite delicately dried the toys and placed them back on the shelves where they belonged. This was quite a contrast with previous sessions, in which Scotty had left the toys out for me to put away.

One memorable Thursday afternoon, Scotty made the single mound that had replaced the other mounds, except that this time he used his fingers to scoop out a small door on the front of the mound. He then selected a small white bear and put him halfway into this doorway—stating "He lives there," and, pointing to the bear, "That's his house." (Internally, I was on my feet clapping, celebrating his use of words. Externally, I remained still, present, and fascinated.) He made the bear's house about four times. After creating each of these sand trays, he retreated to generic play, filling tubs with water and placing a ring of shells around the edges (reminiscent of the earliest stages of his sand trays). He then floated boats in the water and placed sea life in the water, often asking for "grass" to put on the bottom of the sea. I viewed this play as an attempt to symbolize a nurturing environment; perhaps it also reflected some ambivalence about how safe a home on land, like his bear's home, could actually be.

Finally, months after treatment had begun and the bear's home was being intermittently built, Scotty introduced yet another new element into his sand tray story (see Figure 8.4). This sand tray had a different feel

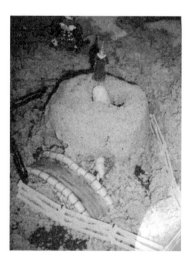

FIGURE 8.4. The bear's castle.

to it; it looked as if Scotty was building a product and wanted to make some statement through this product. He stood back and—to my complete surprise—related the following story:

> *This is the bear's castle [upgraded from a house]. He likes it, and it's safe for him. He has a way out—he can go over the bridge—and then he goes out the doors and plays by himself. The princess watches to make sure he's safe. She watches good. She stays awake all the night long. [He then pointed to a Ninja Turtle, which he had placed behind the princess. He continued his story:] But just in case she gets tired, his [the Ninja Turtle's] job is to make sure that she doesn't fall asleep, but if she does, he's awake and takes care of the bear.*

He told me this story in the final 3 minutes of the session (after the timer bell had rung), and after we took a picture of the tray,[3] he only played with the wet sand tray one other time. From this point on, he chose many other toys to play with (the medical kit, drawing materials, the bop bag, and the dollhouse).

I was intrigued by the fact that Scotty did not refer to his previous wet sand tray play for about a month and a half, so I decided to make some comments to him about the bear's castle. I told Scotty that I had been remembering his bear story. I offered him a piece of paper, some pastels, and line markers, and told him that I wondered what the inside of the bear's castle looked like. He drew a picture, which he took home and showed to his foster mother; Darlene told me that it looked very much like his actual room in their home. He asked that no photo be taken of the picture he made, and it seemed clear that this picture was a special gift for his foster mother (not something he wanted to share with me). This picture (of a child in bed reading) was further evidence that Scotty was feeling more and more secure and "rested," and that his needs for nurturing were being met in his new environment.

During the next session, something quite interesting occurred: Scotty asked me to take the lid off the sand tray, and he poured in water, making the sand damp enough for him to clear away a large circle on the bottom

---

[3] When I explain the use of the sand tray to children, I tell them that once they tell me that they are finished, I usually take pictures of the tray, with their permission. I keep one picture in the office, and they take the other one home. It is rare that children do not give permission to take pictures, and they seem to take great pride in showing their work to parents or caretakers. Some children want to bring their caretakers into the therapy office to view the sand world before it is dismantled. Others prefer to keep the pictures and their experiences to themselves. Parents (and children) are asked to sign permission slips when sand tray pictures are to be shown to professionals or used for publication purposes.

of the tray. Then he proceeded to create a scene in the sand (Figure 8.5), which he described when he was finished:

> *This is my grandmother. She was real nice to the . . . to me. She hugged me when I was scared. She took me out for walks when I was a baby, fed me, and changed my baby diapers. She died, but I remember her. She was nice. She sang to me, humming songs, like you hum.*[4]

This was a sweet memory for Scotty, brought to the surface by my request to draw the inside of his safe castle, followed by his drawing of what was now his new home. In that process of exploring issues of safety, Scotty's earliest memories of his grandmother surfaced, and he was able to "translate" them from abstract to concrete through play. As shown in Figure 8.5, although Scotty was speaking of his grandmother, he chose to use a younger mother figure, even though an older grandmother figure was available to him. It is likely that this scenario was a combination of his longing for his biological mother; his memory of his grandmother as nurturing and safe; the reality of his new (foster) mother, Darlene; and his acknowledgment that even though his grandmother was no longer available to him, he could hold her in his memory, and now could visualize her concretely (since he had created a tangible image in the sand).

Scotty continued in treatment for another 6 months, and his creative energies were now available in a variety of ways. He set up play scenes with motorcycles racing, cars racing, and animals roving a wild forest. Periodically, he would take his games into the dry sand tray, but never the wet tray. He sometimes created environments in the dry sand tray for animals, always making sure that the mother and father animals were nearby and available to the children—who liked to play near, but not always with, the parents. Scotty also responded well to psychoeducational lessons about sexual abuse.

Scotty was eventually adopted by his foster mother, and at a 1-year follow-up phone call, was doing very well; Darlene described him as quite happy and relaxed. I've talked to him myself on the phone from time to time, and he always asks about the play therapy room and wonders if I've still got my sand and the rest of my toys. I heard from the child's social worker that she had received positive reports regarding Scotty's growth and development. Darlene subsequently adopted a 2-

---

[4] Children have consistently pointed out that I hum when I am in sessions with them, and this is something I do without thinking. I have come to recognize that humming is something I associate with nurturing, and I now have wonderful, vivid memories of being held in my grandmother's arms as she hummed to me when I was upset. Those memories were not clear to me prior to child clients' commenting on my humming.

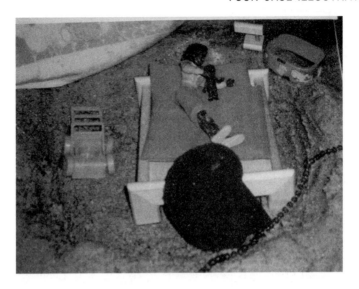

FIGURE 8.5. Inside Scott's castle.

year-old girl and reported that Scotty was helpful and tender with his new sister.

SUMMARY

Scotty was an amazing child exposed to horrific and persistent abuse in his early years. It is a tribute to his resiliency that he was able to utilize treatment, formulate a positive attachment, and learn to trust again. I don't know how children do it! I think it's a miracle that defies explanation. This child eventually learned to view the world as rewarding, in spite of the fact that he had encountered so much pain and suffering when he was little.

My most critical jobs were to provide a safe environment, advocate for safe environments outside the therapy room, and provide consistent and empathic care. I had a reliable and trustworthy treatment team, consisting of a single foster mom (who still remains in my memory as one of the most caring and kind foster parents I have ever met); a social worker who took this case and fought for positive outcomes; a school teacher dedicated to Scotty's comfort level; and myself. Scotty was our focal point, and changing his circumstances became our mission. At one point in the therapy, I felt that we had gathered around Scotty in a little circle and were trying to provide him with a safe enough container for him to grow and thrive, similar to the sand scenarios that appeared in Scotty's later sessions.

My first goal of creating safety was met in the first few months of therapy. Scotty began to see the room (and his therapist) as consistent, nondemanding, and predictable. His fear and anxiety began to decrease as he had new experiences in home, school, and therapy. I was fiercely committed to helping him process his traumas, but I also firmly believed that play therapy would give him the opportunity to externalize and process whatever memories of abuse he needed to understand or tolerate. I was interested in everything he did; I did not come in with hidden agendas of wanting him to work on one thing or another; and I took the pressure off him by accepting his "symptom" of not speaking and by telling him that he did not have to speak in sessions. I also tried to understand and listen to the metaphors in his stories. I helped him expand on those only by giving him an invitation to move from one medium to another (e.g., asking him to draw the inside of the castle). As you remember, he drew the castle's interior, and later constructed a related scene (involving his grandmother) in the sand.

I believe that Scotty exposed himself gradually to difficult memories that had remained overwhelming. He had never been able to process these before, because he had gone from one abusive environment to another and never had a window of time to regroup and begin to feel safety.

Because children have remarkable abilities to survive and thrive by mastering the situations they endure, and at the same time have natural human tendencies to suppress what is painful, art, play, and sand therapies provide them with unique chances for reparative work. This is accomplished at children's individual pace and with built-in safeguards, because once material is exposed, children have yet another choice: to see or not to see what they have created. Their choices may prompt the development of adaptive coping strategies. Clinicians become the containers of truth, witnesses to reality, and holders of images—storing, chronicling, remembering, and reintroducing, often helping clients to elaborate on a reparative motif.

As I have written this chapter, my heart is filled with warmth for this amazing child and his will to live. I can still see that first full smile he gave me. I cherish that wonderful gift.

9

Carla's Search
for Her Lost Mother

REFERRAL INFORMATION

Carla was referred to me by a school social worker, Mr. Biggs, after his initial referral to CPS was not accepted for an investigation. Instead, the CPS worker told Mr. Biggs to seek therapy for the child. If additional concerns arose in therapy, Mr. Biggs was instructed to call back. I listened as Mr. Biggs presented what appeared to be a fairly marginal situation, but the more I learned, the more I felt that CPS needed to be involved.

Carla was 7 years old at the time of the referral. She was a very petite and fragile-looking European American child. Mr. Biggs told me that she had been enrolled in the first grade and had no prior schooling whatsoever. She had never attended preschool or kindergarten, and had only been placed in the first grade because of her age. Academically, she was "catching up" after a rough start. Her teacher described her as "wild and unruly." She had no manners to speak of, seemed uncomfortable with structure of any kind, habitually got out of her chair, and seemed to want to wander around the hallways. Moreover, she spoke whenever she wished, made random statements, and often seemed disoriented and somewhat lost in the classroom environment. The most remarkable feature, according to her teacher, was her physical appearance: Carla smelled bad, wore clothes that barely fit or were inappropriate to the climate, and looked unkempt. She also tried to steal other children's food from their lunch boxes even when it appeared she had sufficient food of her own, and she put her head down on her desk and fell asleep almost daily. Carla's teacher liked the child, but found it troubling that she seemed ill prepared to cope with social demands. Lastly, Carla would often ask whether her mother had come to pick her up, inquire where her mother was, and insist that her father was not her "real" father.

When I listened to Mr. Biggs, I became concerned about neglect, and I opted to call CPS myself before meeting with Carla or her father. At the same time, I thought the situation needed the kind of investigation that I would not provide in therapy. I also hoped that my cordial relationship with the CPS hotline workers might elicit more interest in this case. When I called the hotline, I was happy that a social worker friend of mine answered the phone. She seemed more concerned than her previous colleague, and told me that she would go out to the school and talk to Carla directly. She also said that she would encourage Carla's parent or caretaker to bring the child to therapy, since it sounded as if, at a minimum, the child was anxious.

PSYCHOSOCIAL HISTORY

By the time Carla came to her first appointment, CPS personnel had visited the child at school and found her cooperative and quite candid about her life. The conversation with Carla had sparked an interest in speaking with her primary caretaker, her father, Fred. When they dropped in on Carla and her father, they found the father to be cooperative, honest, and well intentioned. He told them that he and Carla's mother had had a brief relationship but never married, and that the mother had a long-standing drug problem. During her pregnancy she had drunk alcohol, but (to her credit) she had limited the amount she drank, aware that it was hurtful to her unborn child. Fred had become actively involved in Carla's care when she was an infant, but the mother disappeared one day with Carla in tow when Fred was at work. His efforts to locate the mother had failed, since he didn't know anything about her except that she seemed like a drifter with no apparent family ties. The mother had always spoken well about California, where she had some friends, and Fred assumed that she had gone with the child to the West Coast.

A month prior to this referral, Carla was literally dropped on Fred's doorstep by her mother—now a somewhat bewildered, dirty, and sickly woman who had lost weight, continued her drug habit, and seemed detached and anxious to move on. Fred noted that he'd had a 30-minute conversation with the mother "at most." She'd told him that she couldn't handle Carla dragging on her all the time, that she was homeless, and that she needed money. Fred gave her some cash and insisted that she leave Carla with him, although the thought of caring for this small, hyperactive child scared him. The mother did not resist, took the cash, and left a bewildered Carla in his care. He noted that Carla was dirty, seemed hungry, and had no possessions of her own. He immediately called to get her a medical appointment and began the very difficult task of getting to know and help this child. He admitted to checking for a birthmark on her back, to make sure this was the same child he had cared for when she was an infant, and to feeling ambivalent when he found the birthmark.

Fred described that Carla was initially very agitated and talkative. She told her father about sleeping on the street, going to shelters, and never going to school. She said her mother used needles that made her feel better, and had lots of boyfriends who gave her money. The CPS worker felt it prudent to obtain a medical exam with the sexual abuse nurse examiner's program. This exam confirmed that Carla had been sexually and physically abused; that she was malnourished, underweight, and anemic; and that she had a urinary tract infection and a sexually transmitted disease, although her AIDS test was negative. A dental exam revealed gross neglect. Carla often talked about drinking lots of Coke and Pepsi, and initially resisted her father's attempts to give her milk. Her front teeth were rotting out and needed to be pulled. Luckily, there was a second set of teeth coming through, although the dentist thought she might need false teeth in the future. She was quite a sight: very fragile, nervous, bewildered, small, and quite shy and compelling. Luckily for Carla, she elicited great concern from those who met her, and she was gathering a number of professionals committed to meeting whatever needs were identified.

When I asked Fred what he would do if the mother returned to reclaim her child at a later time, Fred reacted immediately: "I won't let her take Carla again. She can barely take care of herself, let alone a little girl." He asked for the name of an attorney and followed up on the referral the next day to begin proceedings to obtain physical and legal custody of Carla. He did this after securing a paternity test that proved he was Carla's father.

Fred was a 44-year-old man at this time who worked in a large factory and had been steadily employed for 20 years. He was a kind and soft-spoken man with few social skills. He had the same droopy, sad eyes that his daughter had. He lived in a large, dark house with his mother, Lilly, a woman in her late 70s, who seemed to have failing health. Fred provided caretaking for his mother in a very matter-of-fact way. As her only child, he never questioned his responsibility to care for his mother. (This caretaking had unwittingly prepared him for taking care of his young child.) He got up in the morning, made his mother breakfast, made their respective lunches, went to work, and returned home at noon to share lunch with his mother. He had no social life to speak of and no one he could truly claim as a close friend. He clearly loved his child, however, and he wanted Carla to have a good childhood, friends, and normality— things he recognized this child had not experienced prior to arriving at his house. He found the nearest neighborhood school and registered Carla there. Fred had been raised by a single mother himself, so the idea of raising Carla alone seemed normal and expectable to him.

CPS personnel found that Fred and his mother were interested in providing a home for Carla, and they believed that with assistance, Fred could learn to provide for his daughter fully. At the same time, they recognized that Carla had special needs (based on her unfortunate first few years of life) and would need special medical services, including a good mental health evaluation and treatment. Since Fred was clearly willing and yet ill equipped to provide for a young child, CPS made a referral for in-home services for 6–9 months to give hands-on help to this unconventional father with a heart of gold. Fred gladly accepted this help, and a number of different in-home workers participated in Carla's case. Carla seemed to attach herself to the first young in-home worker, who stayed approximately 4 months; after that, Carla was friendly but maintained her distance from the in-home workers and other professionals (including me, to a certain extent).

ISSUES SUGGESTED BY PRESENTING PROBLEMS (DECODING OF SYMPTOMS)

Carla had many of the symptoms one would expect from a child with this history. She was not well toilet-trained; she was unable to accept limits; and she did not sleep well at night, often taking a sheet and sleeping on the floor. Her eating habits were unusual: She often ate very quickly and then hoarded some of her food, storing it first in her pockets, and later storing it in different locations around her house. Fred would often discover extra food in her drawers. She was also very hyperalert to loud noises. In addition to her inability to stay in her seat at school, she had very few social skills, so she was shunned by her classmates. She was often fatigued and sleepy. Finally, she constantly asked about her mother— mostly when her mother would come to get her, and who was taking care of the mother. It was as if she expected the mother's return at any moment.

Fred claimed that Carla was doing "okay" at home and seemed to like being with him and his mother. Grandmother Lilly had not yet warmed up to Carla, however, perhaps because she was feeling some-what jealous of the time that Fred now directed toward Carla. Fred also said that Carla was "not very physical" and seemed to freeze when he hugged her. I told Fred early that, given Carla's documented a history of child sexual abuse and her report that the mother's boyfriends had touched and hurt her, she might need extra time to get comfortable with his hugs. I told Fred to inform Carla that daddies often hug and kiss their children on the cheek to say good night, and that he would not hurt her in any way or touch any of her private parts. Fred later commented that she seemed to look right through him the first time he said this, but that over time Carla would repeat the words with him in a soft voice. My hope was that eventually Carla would initiate physical affection with her father, but I knew that this would come only after the father showed himself to be trustworthy.

SYSTEMIC ISSUES

There were obvious systemic issues for this child. In addition to living on the streets with a drug-addicted mother, she had been neglected and physically and sexually abused. The mother had managed to sidestep any systemic intervention to date, and Carla had gone unprotected and mal-treated for most of her young life. It appeared that the mother had availed herself of shelters periodically but had managed to keep her serious prob-lems from professional scrutiny. It was mind-boggling that Carla could have failed to elicit concern from anyone coming into contact with her. I could only imagine that the mother's street savvy had allowed her to keep herself and her daughter "undercover."

Carla's immediate family system had serious limitations, but what Fred and his mother lacked in caretaking skills, he made up for with clear motivation and interest in his child. He was also receptive to any help he could get, and the concrete services provided by in-home services work-ers contributed a lot to his overall parenting acuity. His learning curve was not extremely high, but he made sufficient changes to provide an ad-equate, supportive, and attentive home for Carla. Fred also received help in caring for his mother. Carla participated in an after-school program that she liked better than school, because there were fewer children and less structure.

The in-home workers reported that Fred was capable of mimicking what he was able to observe and learn though role modeling. They also noted that he was "soft" when it came to setting limits for Carla, and that he needed constant reassurance that setting limits was part of being a good parent. I met with Fred in parental coaching sessions, and I maintained close contact with the in-home workers so that I could reinforce their lessons. Eventually we functioned as a professional team for Carla.

TREATMENT PLAN

My plan was to provide individual therapy for Carla. Using a play-based approach, I intended to begin with an extended a developmental assessment, in order to gain an understanding of Carla's inner world. I wanted to provide her with a safe environment and a consistent and empathic therapist with whom she could develop a trusting relationship. In the context of this predictable and consistent therapy relationship, I would assess her strengths, vulnerabilities, idiosyncratic perceptions of her past experiences, and treatment needs, so that I could develop additional treatment goals. Since in-home service workers worked very closely with Fred, I met with him every other month to give him feedback about Carla's therapy progress and to offer any coaching I felt necessary. In addition, the in-home service workers and I kept in touch, exchanging information and ideas, as we got more familiar with Carla and her family.

ASSESSMENT INSTRUMENTS AND TOOLS

I utilized the Child Behavior Checklist (CBCL) to obtain Fred's observations and worries about Carla's behaviors. Her initial CBCL had elevated scales (Anxiety, Thought Disorders). In addition, Fred filled out the Child Sexual Behavior Inventory (CSBI). This instrument showed additional behavioral problems, including Carla's crossing of physical boundaries, talking about explicit sexuality, asking people to touch her private parts, and masturbatory behavior.

Carla was unable or unwilling to do a family play genogram and seemed uninterested in art activities of any kind. She did however, make extensive use of sand therapy as well as puppet play.

OVERALL TREATMENT GOALS

My goals for Carla's treatment were as follows:

Conduct an extended developmental assessment.
Explore Carla's anxiety about her mother, and assess issues of loss and role reversal.

Explore Carla's perceptions, thoughts, and feelings regarding her re-
lationship with her father and grandmother.
Identify and reinforce her adaptive social and coping skills.
Improve her self-image, identity, and self-esteem.
Gain an understanding of issues related to past physical and sexual
abuse.
Provide psychoeducational information regarding physical bound-
aries, appropriate touching, and prevention strategies.

INDICATORS OF TREATMENT PROGRESS

Carla's behaviors could best be described as qualifying for a diagnosis
of PTSD. Given her nightmares, emotionality, intrusive thoughts, reenactment of abuse, hypervigilance, and hyperarousal, it would be critical to ensure that her environment was safe, predictable, and consistent,
and that specific techniques for reducing these symptoms were implemented. Our team approach was to strengthen both the school personnel's and father's abilities to provide nurturing and limit setting to
Carla, so that she would develop a sense of predictability. Toward this
end, the in-home service workers agreed to bolster Fred's parenting
skills, and I agreed to work on the issue of maternal loss and apparent
anxiety associated with the wish for the mother's return. My first recommendation was given to Fred and consisted of his delivering the following message to Carla:

> "I know you are worried about your mommy, but you have to remem-
> ber that she is a grownup and will take care of herself. She has gone to
> live in California, and she won't be coming back here. Grandma Lilly
> and I are going to build a home for you . . . a home that is safe and a
> home you can count on. You're going to live with us, go to school, and
> do things that other little girls your age do . . . Even if Mommy comes
> back sometime, she'll only come back to visit. You won't go back to
> live with her, because you, Grandma Lilly, and I are a family now."

I helped Fred practice this message, and the coaching paid off. Both
he and Grandma Lilly (once the grandmother got over her initial jeal-
ousy) reinforced this message constantly, and the results were positive:
Eventually Carla seemed better able to shift her attention to the present
and began to ask fewer questions about her mother. In spite of the fact
that her verbal questions slowed down and she seemed less preoccupied
with her mother's absence (e.g., she paid less attention to cars pulling up
to the house or the phone ringing), her play reflected a deep and persis-

tent concern that I recognized as a deep pattern of role reversal (she was acutely concerned with the question of who was caring for her mother, now that they were separated).

TIME FRAME

I expected to complete my extended developmental assessment in 3 months' time. I then hoped to turn my attention to the goals I had identified prior to beginning treatment, as well as those included after my getting to know Carla and prioritizing her therapeutic needs. I anticipated that this would be a long-term case, and the initial funding was for 6-month intervals (the treatment lasted for three funding periods, or 18 months). When termination occurred, it was due to Carla's treatment progress, not to funding concerns.

PLAY TECHNIQUES

I believed that Carla would benefit from utilizing the standard play therapy equipment in my office. At the same time, given her past experience, I thought it useful to include a few more items: a sleeping bag, campfire, grocery store cart, miniature foods, and little blankets. I also added some drug paraphernalia, including a small plastic hypodermic needle, a rubber hose, and pill bottles.

Because I believed that Carla had suffered traumatic stressors while living on the street with her drug-addicted mother, I found it important to offer her ample opportunities to do literal acting out with toys. I am never sure ahead of time whether children will move toward engaging in posttraumatic play; however, I find that anticipating and introducing literal symbols (particularly when there is a documented history of trauma) may relax defenses and allow for symbolic processing (consciously or unconsciously motivated).

THERAPY SESSIONS

When I saw Carla for the first time, she reminded me of the title character from the Broadway show *Annie*, with her too-tight pants and her outfit as a whole in colors and fabrics that had little relationship to each other. She moved slowly toward me, gave me her hand, and seemed ready to go with me wherever I wished. Her father said, "This is the doctor I told you about. She's got a nice room with lots of toys." We came upstairs, and Carla separated from Fred too easily for my comfort. I allowed Fred to wait outside the play therapy office, and Carla seemed to look around with curiosity and slight trepidation: "Are you going to give me a shot?" "No," I reassured her, "I'm not *that* kind of doctor!" I explained to her that I was a doctor who would meet with her once a week and get to know her; we would "sometimes play and sometimes talk." I showed her around the room, pointing out all the different activities. I told her that this was her time, and she could decide what she wanted to do.

She was cautious as she put her hands in one of the sand trays. She preferred the rust-colored sand and asked if she could play with it. I adjusted the placement of the tray so that it was comfortable for her to play with it, and thus began our therapy relationship. She enjoyed burying her hands in the sand and surprising me when they emerged suddenly. I was reminded of the fact that her mother had a history of appearing and disappearing and surprising her. I made a note that she might already be using play therapy symbolically. Carla loosened up as she did this activity, and her little body appeared less tense. However, she still reacted to every noise in the room—the clock, the heater going on and off, and noises from other rooms. She was able to ask about these noises, which I thought was positive. I would reassure her for the first 6 months about the noises in the room.

The first four sessions all proceeded in similar fashion. She always looked around first and even picked up some of the toys that were displayed, but she always came back to the sand and her hide-and-seek behavior. She asked me to mimic her hands, and she put a surprised look on her face when my hands rose out of the sand. I would comment, "You're surprised to see my hands. They were covered with sand." "They're hiding," she said, and added, "We have to find them." She then shifted her attention to finding missing things, and would take small crystals and bury them in the sand. The game consisted of her telling me to cover my eyes, her placing the crystals in the sand, and her supervising my retrieval of each crystal.

At about the sixth session, she found some miniatures that became the staples of her play: Winnie-the-Pooh, Tigger, and Roo. She had never read the A. A. Milne books or seen the Disney films featuring these characters, and I told her what their names were. She was extremely fond of Roo, always taking great care to leave her (Carla had decided that Roo was a "her") somewhere safe before the end of a session (in a tissue, in a little box, in a nest). I began to believe that Carla was identifying with Roo as a motherless child. She had asked early on, "Where is Roo's mommy?" (perhaps noticing that Roo was a baby and that the other two characters were of different species—a bear and a tiger). I told her that it seemed Roo's mother was nowhere to be found, and from that point on she would enter the room and ask about Roo's mom. (At this time I thought about buying Roo's mom, Kanga, since she was not yet part of my collection, but I believed that it would be more beneficial to allow Carla to process her loss issues in this way.)

I concluded my assessment with a clear belief that Carla was processing her loss issues symbolically and that she was an excellent play therapy candidate. I believed that we were forging a good relationship, and I decided that I would continue my nondirective stance and active observation, along with intermittent coaching of her father and collaboration with the in-home workers. Since Carla had introduced the theme of a lost mother and a searching baby, I felt we were on our way to helping her with her relational issues of abandonment.

Within the first few months, therefore, Carla had established a routine; she had chosen projective symbols; and she had developed a comfort with me as the clinician and with the play therapy office. She began to sleep through the night after a good-night ritual with her father and grandmother. Fred had begun reading to her at night almost as soon as she moved in, and although at first she was distracted and uninterested, she eventually began listening, asking questions about the stories, enjoying the stories, and asking for them to be read. (I purposely held off on suggesting Milne's *Winnie-the-Pooh* books, because I wanted her to have as open an identification with these characters as possible.)

Not only was Roo an important and heavily utilized symbol object for Carla, but Winnie himself became quite relevant when she dubbed him "Roo's dad." She said, "He's nice and he can take care of Roo. He's warm and . . . [in a soft voice] he won't hurt her or touch her privates." Winnie had become Fred in her eyes, and to be honest, I hardly ever look at Fred any more without seeing his remarkable similarity to Winnie-the-Pooh.

The play soon became more active and complex. Each week Carla came in, selected her toys, and set up stories, sometimes in the sand tray and sometimes on the floor. During one of the sessions when Roo went searching for her mother, Carla moved into a different part of the room and found the puppet bin. She abandoned Roo and took all the animals out of the bin. There she found a mother kangaroo, a joey that lived in the mother's pouch, a mother sheep and her lamb, and a mother bird (who had a worm in her mouth) with a nest and three baby birds. (She purposely chose the blue birds to match the mother's color, setting aside the three brown baby birds.)

For the next 3 months, Carla's play continued to be focused on babies looking for their mothers. At the end of each session, I would state, "The babies keep looking for their mommies." "Yep," she would say, "next time we'll see what's what!" (one of her father's favorite expressions). Her demeanor was changing: She was more cheerful and assertive, and her voice was a little louder—she was no longer whispering, but certainly not shouting either.

One Monday afternoon, the play shifted when the joey instructed the other animal babies to "cross the highway" and follow her. The mothers had been placed behind a big chair every week as Carla began her play. This week, the joey crossed the highway, climbed the mountain (chair), and looked over the top of the mountain to find the mothers huddled together. "Kids, kids, come here," she announced, "I think I've found our mothers!" I brought the other kids closer (as she instructed me to do), and we all climbed to look over the top of the chair. "Are you sure it's the mommies?" I asked. "Of course, can't you see? It's our mommies down there . . . they must have fallen off the mountain. We better go look and see if they're hurt." Carla pulled aside the chair and with the most gentle hands you can imagine, her joey puppet on one or two fingers, she grabbed the mother kangaroo and brought her out from behind the chair. In a somber voice she reported, "She's a little bit hurt . . . we might have to call 911." She guided me to call 911, and I dialed a toy phone and asked her what to say. "Tell them someone needs help and to *come fast!*" I repeated the message with the same loud and urgent tone in my voice. Carla held the mother in her lap, stroking her head, as she waited for the ambulance to arrive. She then gave the mother kangaroo and joey to me to hold and went into emergency mode. She got the medical equipment; put on rubber gloves, a surgical mask, and a stethoscope; and came over with a play hypodermic needle in her hand. "I hear there's been a problem," she said. "Where's the patient?" "She's over here, Doctor. We think she fell off the mountain," I replied. Carla, dressed as the doctor, looked at the kangaroo's ears, eyes, and mouth. She listened to her chest and back, asking her to take a deep breath. She shook her head and mumbled, "Oh, oh, oh, oh." Finally she looked up at me and said, "I have the perfect medicine to cure this mommy kangaroo." She gave the kangaroo a shot and quietly said to her, "I know this will hurt a little, but it's full of good medicine, not bad medicine, and it will make you feel better soon." The session was nearing an end. Carla grabbed the mother kangaroo, stuck the joey in her pouch, and said, "Sleep now, Mommy, so that tomorrow you can take care of your baby."

The following weeks, the lamb's and the baby birds' mothers were rescued and given medicine in the same way. Carla asked to make a "home" for these reunited mothers and children, and we did an arts and crafts project in which she decorated a large box on the outside, and made a soft pillowy floor inside for the mother animals and their children to live on.

Once this play occurred, Carla seemed more focused on her school and social activities, and used less symbolic work. She made sand scenarios that seemed to represent more of a fantasy world at times, and forests with animal families at other times. One day we had the following conversation:

CARLA: Do you think my mom will ever come find me?

THERAPIST: Your mother lives in California now, so I can't answer that question. (*Pause*) She might come to visit someday, but I don't think she'll be well enough to take care of you all the time.

CARLA: She has a big problem with drugs.

THERAPIST: How do you know that?

CARLA: My dad told me but I already knew. . . . She put bad medicine in with a needle. She put it in between her toes and hands. She had big bruises on her arms.

THERAPIST: How sad that some mommies have problems with drugs and can't take care of their babies.

CARLA: Yeah. One of my friends at school lives with her grandma too, because her mom drinks too much whiskey.

THERAPIST: Yeah, it happens. (*Pause*) How do you feel when you think of your mom now?

CARLA: I can't remember her a lot . . . I think she was gone a lot and sick a lot.

THERAPIST: Oh. Do you get feelings when you think of her?

CARLA: I just can't remember very much.

THERAPIST: Okay, sounds like you can't remember much about your mom right now.

CARLA: No, never! I can't remember her face.

I decided to have a directive family therapy session to address this issue of Carla's loss of memory about her mother. I thought it might be useful if Carla and her father could talk about their memories of her mother and do some kind of closure ritual, since Carla now seemed more prepared to acknowledge the loss and since she seemed to have given up her role of caring for the mother at this point (having nurtured the mother through her play). Up to this time, Fred had felt very uncomfortable discussing Carla's mother because of his anger at the mother, which would become visible immediately. I cautioned Fred to stay as neutral as possible, and he followed the direction well.

I also prepared Fred to participate in this session by asking him to bring whatever pictures he had of Carla's mother (he had one). I gave Fred and Carla a large piece of construction paper, and I asked them to put the picture in the middle of the sheet and then start thinking about any and all memories that they had. I gave them a lot of pictures that had been cut out from magazines (my collage pictures). I asked them to go through and pick whatever reminded them of the mother. Carla found a pair of shoes and said, "Mom's shoes were always broken." Then the father found a bottle of whiskey and stated, "Mom used to drink too much." Fred also found pictures of the sea, a California mountainside, a folk singer, and a German shepherd dog. He told Carla how these pictures reminded him of Carla's mother. Carla found pictures of spaghetti ("Mom's favorite food"), a Denny's restaurant ("where we asked for money"), and ribbons ("Mom used to put ribbons in my hair.") Slowly but surely, the piece of construction paper was filled up with pictures that represented memories of the mother. I asked them to think of a title for the picture, and they agreed on "What We Remember about Carla's Mom." They both felt proud of their accomplishment, and I remarked, "Looks like there's lots of happy and sad memories about Mom." "Yep," Carla said as she put the sheet of construction paper under her arm and started to walk away. "You help me, Dad," she said, and asked him to hold one end of the sheet as they walked out.

Sexual abuse issues surfaced only in passing during the treatment. A few times Carla used boy and girl figures to indicate kissing. Toward the end of therapy, I invited Fred and Carla to watch a videotape called *Three Kinds of Touches* (Pennsylvania Coalition against Rape, n.d.), and we reviewed appropriate physical boundaries. It is likely that her sexual abuse had occurred at such a young age that she didn't have conscious memory of the event(s). At the same time, I talked to Fred about behaviors that might signal a problem as Carla got older. Fred had learned how to talk to Carla about "too-tight hugging" and about appropriate privacy. Carla had initially undressed in the living room and gone to the bathroom with the door open. She had altered those behaviors as Fred and his mother were able to set appropriate limits.

After discharge, the 6-month follow-up was positive. Carla was doing well at school; she had few problem behaviors; she was more socially adept; and she had several good friends and playmates.

SUMMARY

Carla was a small, frail-looking child who had suffered a great deal in her young life. Her drug-addicted mother had been homeless for years and yet somehow managed to avoid any attention from social services until Carla was about 5 years of age. At that point, Carla had lived in several shelters and had been both physically and sexually abused (as a subsequent examination documented). The mother would often leave her unattended or in the care of other street people; her efforts to be a good mother were overcome by her drug addiction. Recognizing her own limitations, the mother eventually brought Carla to the child's father, Fred, and disappeared.

Fred was a kind and sweet man, ill prepared but willing to take responsibility for his daughter. He evolved into a very stable parent and made remarkable efforts to learn from those assigned to teach him parenting skills. He brought Carla to therapy consistently and willingly, and he constantly sought guidance in order to reassure his child and give her the best opportunities he could. We met occasionally for coaching sessions, and he received help from in-home workers that bolstered his parenting skills significantly.

Carla's therapy was mostly nondirective and based on her utilization of play therapy. She immediately chose symbolic objects to represent her acute concern for the safety of her mother. Her play consistently showed her preoccupation with "finding" her mother and an underlying concern that the mother was in need of help. Because Carla's mother had established a role reversal, Carla had often been in charge of making sure that her mother was clean, healthy, and fed. Carla was now intensely worried that no one was taking care of her mother.

The major theme of her play was a "search for mother," which eventually resulted in an emergency rescue and in subsequent medical care. These two events were enacted in turn with a mother kangaroo and her joey, a mother sheep and her lamb, and a mother bird and her three babies in a nest. It was probably in the last component of this play—the provision of medical care (and "good medicine")—that Carla symbolically did what she could for her missing mother, and in so doing was able to let go of her anxiety.

In addition to coaching Carla's father from time to time about what to say about her mother and how to continue to set good limits (e.g., concerning what she wore and whether she combed her hair), I had a session with Carla and her father that allowed them to jointly memorialize Carla's mother.

This child was tremendously resilient and resourceful. She elicited a positive response from those who met her; initially it was caretaking, but later it moved to warmth and interest. Carla had experienced great distress in her life, and the predominant theme had been survival. Her mother had often placed her in harm's way, but had also nurtured her to the best of her limited abilities.

10

Danger in the Backyard

REFERRAL INFORMATION

The police called late in the evening, concerned about a 5-year-old European American girl, Jessica R., who had been abused in her backyard—ostensibly by a 12- or 13-year-old boy unknown to the family. The caller simply said, "The mom is a wreck, and reporters are gathered outside her front door . . . she's talking to them, and she's going to be on the morning TV news." The police officer added that there was no penetration, but it appeared that "there was oral cop and fondling." Jessica's mother had already inquired about counseling for her daughter, and I scheduled an intake appointment for the mother right away. Mrs. R. indeed sounded distraught on the phone, noting, "Jessica seems clingy and nervous."

PSYCHOSOCIAL HISTORY

The mother was a 39-year-old European American female who was in her second marriage. She and her husband lived with Jessica and with 16-year-old Piper (Mrs. R.'s daughter by her first marriage). Piper had virtually no contact with her birth father and seemed uninterested in establishing a relationship with Mr. R., often complaining that he was "a weirdo." Jessica and her older sister shared a positive, nurturing, and warm relationship, however, and the mother remarked that "Piper acts like this happened to her. She's furious and blames me for not watching Jessica well enough." The maternal and paternal grandparents were out of the picture and lived in other states. I asked the mother whether she had let the grandparents know about what had occurred, and she noted, "They would just blame me too." The mother had lived in her current home for approximately 8 years, and Jessica had attended kindergarten for 4 months without incident.

During the intake appointment, Mrs. R. described the events surrounding Jessica's molestation as best she could. She cried throughout this interview, clearly distraught by this sudden, unexpected life stressor. She seemed consumed with guilt that she had "let this happen." She described always watching her daughter through the kitchen window when Jessica was playing outside. There were woods behind the play area, and the mother always insisted that Jessica stay close to the house: "She knew she wasn't supposed to go into the woods unless her dad or sister or me were with her." I could see her desperate attempts to place the blame— first on herself for not seeing someone approach Jessica, and then on Jessica for going into the woods and breaking house rules.

Apparently the phone rang while Mrs. R. watched Jessica and washed dishes. She went to answer a call and had to go find her purse to give a credit card number to the salesperson on the phone. "I should have told them to call back. I shouldn't have answered the phone . . . I couldn't have been gone more than 5 minutes." In that time, a teenage boy approached Jessica, took her hand, and led her into the woods. When mother came back to the window, she couldn't see Jessica. She spent another 5 or 10 minutes going to her nearby neighbors and asking whether they knew where Jessica had gone. "I knew right away something was wrong . . . she never goes off by herself." The mother then started yelling into the woods—a sound that clearly scared off the boy—and Jessica appeared in view without her underpants and with a scared look on her face. The mother asked what had happened, and Jessica said, "A big boy touched my privates." Mrs. R. picked her up and rushed to the police station. She called her husband from the police station, but he was not available by phone. Piper, likewise, was unavailable on her pager. The mother reported having a "frantic time" and feeling so worried that something horrible had happened. Finally she felt reassured when police told her that it appeared that the boy had run away and hadn't had a chance to "go further" than he did. The mother seemed to focus on whether or not there had been penile penetration and was very relieved to hear there hadn't. When I asked the mother whether the police had told her the specifics of what had occurred, she noted, "They said that he exposed himself to her, had her touch and kiss his penis, and put his hand on her private parts." I did not press for more information and obtained a signed release to talk to the police officer in charge of the investigation, Sergeant Dreiker.

In the course of the intake session, I discovered that Jessica was a happy child—friendly, bright, and doing very well at school. By contrast, the mother reported "typical problems" with her daughter Piper, as well as some "distance that I hope she grows out of." In addition, Mrs. R. kept hinting at her husband's unavailability and extreme work habits. For example, when she told me that she couldn't reach him right away, she added, "That's nothing new, believe me." He had refused to come to the intake session, saying that he "could not take time off from work." When I asked about his availability to come to future sessions, she replied, "I wouldn't count on it."

The mother noted that her husband was very different from herself: "We couldn't be more different if we tried. I'm a wreck and teary and scared, while he's Mr. Cool, Calm, and Collected." When I asked the mother if she knew how Mr. R. was feeling, she said, "I'm sure he's upset and angry at the kid [i.e., the teenage boy]. He loves Jessie a lot, but you'd never know it to see him."

I rearranged my schedule to see Jessica immediately—partly because the mother was so distraught, and partly because it sounded as though the child had been through a very scary experience. The mother's description of her initial concerns indicated that Jessica could be experiencing acute anxiety symptoms.

ISSUES SUGGESTED BY PRESENTING PROBLEMS

The mother's initial concerns, as she had indicated on the phone, were Jessica's "clinginess" and "nervousness." This event had just occurred, so there had been little time to observe Jessica's reactions in more detail. Mrs. R. described the clinginess as Jessica's "hanging on" to her mother and not wanting to be left alone, and she described the nervousness as Jessica's being "jumpy . . . she jumps at any little noise; she's looking around the room all the time." I explained to the mother that it would be expectable for Jessica to be startled by the events of the last few days. Not only had she been (allegedly) sexually abused by a stranger in her backyard, but she had been interviewed by the police, and she had been taken to the hospital for a medical exam. (Apparently Jessica started crying uncontrollably at the hospital, and the nurse decided to defer the exam to a later date.) In addition, there had been lots of strangers on her doorsteps, as well as many phone calls and visitors from the neighborhood.

SYSTEMIC ISSUES

The emergency nature of this referral, as well as the mother's initial distress in the intake session, did not allow for extensive exploration of systemic issues. It appeared to me that Jessica's mother was in crisis mode and looking for guidance, and I made a particular note of the mother's statements about the father's unavailability. The larger system was in full action as the police force continued its investigation and apparently narrowed the field quickly to a suspect in a nearby neighborhood. Sergeant Dreiker, the police officer with whom I spoke, told me he would be back in touch as soon as they knew more. Fortunately, he was a sensitive and well-trained person, who had taken his time interviewing Jessica and her mother. The mother felt that the interview with Sergeant Dreiker had gone very well, and she was glad they had been able to ask their questions right away. "She's so young," Mrs. R. noted, "that it's better if they ask her about this while she still remembers."

Mrs. R. commented on her husband's general remoteness and his absence from the intake session in particular as "typical." She noted that they had been having problems for a while and seemed to have very little to say to each other any more. She stated that she felt completely without support from him, but on some level she seemed no longer surprised at his passivity.

PARENTAL COACHING

During the intake session with the mother, I encouraged her to make an appointment with her current therapist (whom she hadn't seen for almost 6 months); I asked her to try to talk with her husband to see whether they could face this challenge together; and I coached her a little about what to say and not to say to Jessica about the abuse. I told Mrs. R. that there was a group available for nonoffending mothers, but when she found out that most of the parents had incest in their families, she declined the invitation to attend.

I also told the mother that I would meet with her separately so that I could check on how Jessica was doing at home, and I told her to call me and let me know of any changes that might occur in the next few days or weeks. I reassured Mrs. R. that I worked with many children who had experienced sexual abuse, and I felt confident that we would be able to find out how Jessica was doing and prepare a response that would help. The mother left a little more calm than she came in, grateful that I would see her daughter the next day.

TREATMENT PLAN AND GOALS

My initial plan was to conduct a shorter developmental assessment with special attention to Jessica's reactions to her sexual abuse. It became clear quickly that Jessica was experiencing anxiety, and I worked with the mother to focus her energies on creating a safe external environment. I worked with Jessica and her mother in parallel interactive fashion: Often I learned from Jessica's play about family functioning, and met with the mother to ascertain clarity, give directives, and facilitate Jessica's restoration of safety with her family and in her home. (These strategies are described in greater detail under "Therapy Sessions," below.)

ASSESSMENT INSTRUMENT AND TOOLS

I asked Mrs. R. to fill out the CBCL, and she returned it to me a few weeks later. It revealed that within the first few weeks since the abuse, Jessica had developed several symptoms of PTSD, including nightmares, emotionality, intrusive flashbacks, and repetitive talking about the "bad woods." Further assessment was conducted through observations of Jessica's distinctive play, particularly her scenarios she constructed in a sand box.

INDICATORS OF TREATMENT PROGRESS

My immediate goals were to understand Jessica's experience of her abuse and to decrease the symptomatic behaviors reported to me. In particular, I was interested in decreasing signs of anxiety and assisting Jessica to regain her sense of security and safety. Specifically, I looked for the following as signs of treatment progress: increasing autonomy, less clinginess, fewer nightmares, a return to prior activities (e.g., playing outside by herself), and less incessant talking about the woods.

TIME FRAME

Given the fact that the reported abuse consisted of a single incident, as well as the remarkable qualities Jessica exhibited in our first session (see below) and her positive relationship with her mother and sister, I anticipated that therapy would be short-term (in this case, about 4 months). Of course, this projection was based on initial impressions and did not take into account other variables that can, and do, intrude into people's lives.

PLAY TECHNIQUES

Nondirective play therapy allows children to self-select their activities. Some children may be experiencing acute and obvious stressors and may not be able to access symbolic language or use play to externalize or address their concerns, so it may be necessary to "tickle the defenses" by utilizing gradually more directive strategies. As I have mentioned in Chapter Two, some children may require or demand directive, verbal strategies to help them resolve questions, to alleviate symptoms, and to provide a corrective experience.

Jessica was completely committed to building sand trays, and in so doing pinpointed internal shifts in her perceptions, thoughts, and feelings. She was definitely capable of making herself clear in her play, seemed to process material through right-hemisphere activity, relaxed herself, and gained mastery through gradual exposure and "processing" of her play. In addition, the mother was devoted to her daughter, responded well to all my suggestions, and participated fully in her child's recovery process.

THERAPY SESSIONS

In what follows, I describe a remarkable journey for a very young child exposed to a sudden, unexpected, frightening event that challenged her sense of safety and security. Even as I chronicle this case today, I marvel in the human capacity for healing and restoration of full, glorious functioning.

Jessica was very shy at our first meeting and clung to her mother's legs. The mother maneuvered herself quite well and practically carried Jessica in. I showed Jessica the play therapy office, as I had shown it to the mother the day before. Her eyes widened, but she didn't let go of her mother for at least 10 minutes. At the end of that time, she came over to touch the soft white sand in one of the sand trays. I had been touching the sand, sifting it, and commenting on how soft it felt. I invited the mother to put her hand in, and she had; she also noted that Jessica had a sandbox in her backyard, but that the sand was not as soft as the sand in my tray. Once Jessica touched the sand, her demeanor changed. She seemed to get completely absorbed in building a scenario in the sand, using miniatures available in the room. The mother faded into the background and I invited her to sit on a nearby couch, which she did. Jessica never looked up again until a sand scenario was complete.

Jessica's first sand scenario was quite a wonder to behold. This first

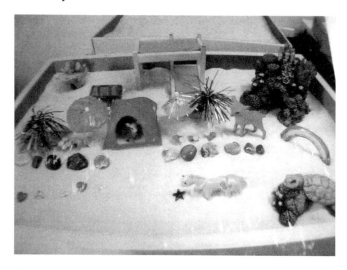

FIGURE 10.1. Jessica's first sand tray.

sand tray, and her subsequent play, provided sufficient information for me to surmise her internalized thoughts and feelings about her abuse (see Figure 10.1).

Jessica first placed a tent almost in the center of the tray. Inside the tent she placed a fawn, choosing to put the mother doe nearby, "watching" the baby deer. In this very small movement, she expressed her need for shelter or protection (the tent), as well as her mixed feelings about her mother's presence and absence (in other words, the mother was watching but was sufficiently removed that she might not see). In addition, she put a little row of rocks and crystals in front of the tent, which served as a barrier. At the back of the tent (upper third of the sand tray), she put her bedroom (bed bunks), and in the front third, she placed an object from a fish tank that appeared to be a mountain filled with openings. My interpretation was that Jessica was referencing the dangers of the woods and being taken into a dark place where she did not feel safe. This scenario was very organized, and she spent quite a bit of time placing each small object just so. In this process, she calmed herself, got comfortable, and allowed herself to experience her mother's watching from the couch. She looked up when she finished her sand scene and exclaimed, "This is fun. Can I play over here?" I told her that she could do anything she wanted in this room, and what she did or said was for her to decide. She went to a Playmobil structure of a hospital with hospital rooms, medical equipment, ambulance, doctors, and medicine. She then continued to reveal what was on her mind (see Figure 10.2).

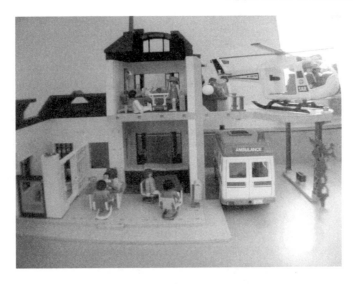

FIGURE 10.2. Jessica's hospital.

In her hospital scenario, Jessica first put a baby and a little girl in one of the hospital rooms. A doctor was also placed in the room, and she noted, "The doctor is taking care of them." I simply repeated what she had said, not wanting to interrupt her process by asking questions. She then carefully put little bottles of medicine on a table next to the doctor, and put an IV bottle next to the little girl. Finally, she put a "mother" in the room and stated that the mother was "visiting." She then went to an elevator that moved up and down between the first and second floors of the hospital (Figure 10.3). She filled the elevator with small people figures, and then noted, "These are the policemen who are making sure no one gets in there to hurt them." Again, I listened and repeated what Jessica had said.

Finally, Jessica used another small room in the hospital some children think of as a jail because it has bars. She put a "bad guy" in that room, calling him that, and then brought a toilet into that room. "Ha, ha," she said, "he's going to the bathroom and everybody can see him . . . ha, ha!" "I see," I said, "he's going potty and everyone can see him . . . What are the people thinking?" I asked, finally taking a chance to ask a question. "They're laughing at him because he's bad, and now everybody sees him going potty."

I was completely fascinated by this child's capacity to make use of play. In the hospital play, she had selected two children, a girl and a baby, and made them "patients" (Figure 10.4). On some level, Jessica was iden-

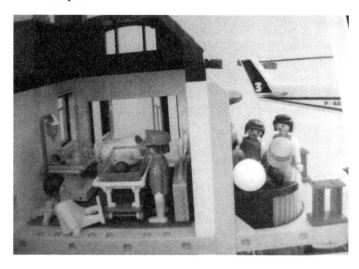

FIGURE 10.3. Jessica's protectors.

tifying her injury and need for help. She had placed the patients in a hospital, so help was accessible and available to them. In addition, she had put protectors near the room (police officers). Finally, in the second sand tray scenario, she had identified a "bad guy" who appeared to be experiencing humiliation by having his private parts exposed. It was possible to

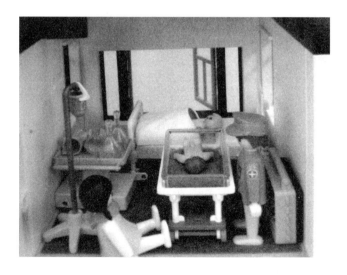

FIGURE 10.4. Jessica's "girl" and "baby."

interpret this "bad guy" in two ways: as the person who had abused her, or as an embodiment of her own self-reproach for being a "bad girl" and going into the woods, breaking the family rules. However, all interpretations were tentative at this point. The important thing was that the choices Jessica made reflected her ability to externalize her concerns through play and appeared to be quite literal depictions of her recent experiences. I often associate this ability to use play literally with post-traumatic play.

The mother had already signed permission for me to take pictures of Jessica's work. When Jessica finished her play and I told her it was time to stop, I mentioned that sometimes I take pictures of what children make when they play, and I asked her if this was okay. She nodded her head, and I took several pictures of her sand tray and hospital play. However, she didn't ask for the pictures in our next session, so I did not provide them. In Jessica's case, I showed her all her pictures during termination, and she never expressed an interest in taking the pictures home.

When Jessica left the session, she seemed physically more relaxed. She skipped out, told her mother she "liked coming here," asked when she could come back, and smiled at me when I shook her hand and told her I had enjoyed meeting her. She had spent 45 minutes setting up the two scenarios—one in the sand, and one in the Playmobil hospital. I had learned a lot from my first meeting with Jessica, and she will always remain in my memory as one of my favorite sand therapy clients.

In subsequent therapy sessions, Jessica continued to construct sand scenarios involving a young baby; a little girl; an attentive, nurturing mother; and an absent father, indicated by an empty chair next to a computer. The longer the play continued, the easier it was to understand that Jessica was showing herself in two ways: as the regressed baby who had been injured, and as the "big girl" who could handle things. Throughout the process, the baby girl was taken care of, nurtured, protected, and encouraged. More and more, the big girl took center stage, eventually becoming the central character.

As the scenarios with the family group shifted over time, I became aware from Jessica's comments and invented dialogues concerning the absent father figure that Mr. and Mrs. R. might have reached a breaking point in their relationship. I asked Mrs. R. about her marriage, and she confirmed that she and her husband had indeed separated and that Mr. R. had moved out of the family home. Although regular visitations with her father had been scheduled for Jessica, Mr. R. was not always consistent about keeping to the schedule, or about keeping other promises he had made to Jessica when he did appear. Jessica continued to work

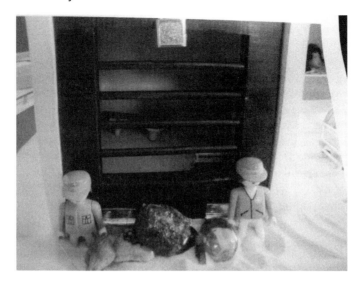

FIGURE 10.5. Jessica's jailed mother.

through these disappointments, and her other feelings concerning the parental separation, as her sandplay evolved.

In a different sand scenario, Jessica provided a very important clue about her feelings toward her mother. This scenario coincided with a call from the mother regarding Jessica's oppositional behavior. Mrs. R. said that Jessica had started talking back, stomping her feet, disobeying, and generally behaving in atypical ways. In this sand scenario, Jessica placed the little box with bars (the "jail") that she had used in an earlier session. She placed guards outside the box and reinforced the outside with rocks (appearing to strengthen the security). When I looked inside the box, she had the little toilet she had used in her earlier hospital play, but had placed the mother doe in the jail (Figure 10.5). My interpretation of this was that Jessica might be feeling angry at her mother for not protecting her. In the following session, I noted that I had seen the mother deer in the jail and asked how come the mom was in jail. Jessica firmly stated, "She was bad . . . she didn't take care of her baby." "Really?" I asked. "The mom didn't take care of her baby?" "No," Jessica said, "and her baby is mad at her and won't let her out until she says she's sorry." I took my lead from Jessica and called Mrs. R. for a coaching session. I encouraged her to talk to Jessica about the abuse and to apologize to her for having looked away long enough for Jessica to get hurt. The mother reported later that the conversation went very well and Jessica simply said, "It's okay to say you're sorry, Mommy . . . sometimes mommies can make mistakes." Mrs. R. reported that Jessica's behaviors went back to normal shortly after this conversation.

Jessica's last sand scenario was very interesting (Figure 10.6). She had a river going down the center of the tray and put the little baby inside a boat. One family (parents and two girls) were on one side of the tray, and they were waving goodbye to the little baby in the boat, who was going down the river to be met by a new family. I believe this was Jessica's way of bidding farewell to the injured baby, restoring herself as a more competent, confident older girl (she had just turned 6).

Jessica is 10 years old today, and her mother calls from time to time to brag about how well she's doing. The mother and Jessica have since moved into an apartment complex; Piper has left for college; Mr. and Mrs. R.'s divorce is final; and the mother has a satisfying long-term relationship with a man whom Jessica likes well. Jessica's father remains a part of her life, and the mother feels that Jessica views her father "realistically" and is happy to see him when she does, but has lower expectations than before that he will keep the promises he makes to her.

Jessica remembers that a boy touched her private parts, but hardly ever brings it up any more. This event is not highlighted to others. The mother once reported that while Jessica and a friend were watching an after-school special about child sexual abuse, Jessica told her friend, "That happened to me when I was a baby . . . the boy got in big trouble!" Her friend did not inquire further, and Jessica did not volunteer more information.

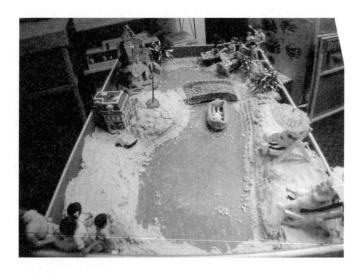

FIGURE 10.6. Jessica's termination sand tray.

The mother also once raised this issue when the school sent home materials to review on child safety. However, this event has gradually taken its place among a series of other stressful experiences Jessica has had: her parents' divorce, a good friend's fatal car accident, and changing schools.

SUMMARY

Jessica R. had an acute single incident of child sexual abuse that was temporarily disorienting. She had acute symptoms of fear and anxiety, and exhibited behaviors that reflected her temporary loss of control. The abuse was perpetrated by a stranger whom Jessica never saw again. It was easier for her to think of him as a "boy who did bad things," because she had no preexisting relationship with him. On the other hand, the fact that this abuse occurred literally in her backyard, while her mother was ostensibly watching her, left Jessica feeling insecure and vulnerable. The fact that her mother had "been there and not been there" produced conflictual emotions for Jessica, and she found these difficult to negotiate or express; thus they produced acting-out behaviors (although these were short-lived and were resolved after a few conversations between mother and daughter).

In addition to the sexual abuse, her parents' subsequent separation linked the abuse closely in time to her father's apparent rejection—quite complicated experiences for such a young child. Moreover, her sister's departure for college, her change of environment, and the loss of a good friend could have conspired to overwhelm Jessica's coping abilities. However, Jessica was very resilient and drew on well-established and nurturing primary relationships, and these anchored and buffered her well.

Jessica remains one of the most intriguing children I've ever met. Her ability to access and utilize healing mechanisms has few parallels in my experience. In addition, her mother's commitment to helping Jessica was complete and unlimited.

Most importantly, Jessica was able to externalize her fears and concerns, to address them by mobilizing and manipulating her play, and to benefit clearly from strong familial support. She engaged in posttraumatic play with abandon, and the results were clear: Her anxiety decreased; her clinginess stopped; she restored a sense of control and mastery; and she was able to draw upon internal and external sources of help to cope with other challenges in her life.

11

The Witch, the Baby, and the Bug

REFERRAL INFORMATION

Nicole was a 4-year-old African American girl who was referred to the ACTS by the DFS for an extended developmental assessment (see Chapter Two). She had been recently removed from her biological father's home because of his inability to provide safe and adequate care for her. At the time of the referral, DFS was in the process of investigating the father. There was a clear possibility that Nicole might have been sexually abused by her father, based on past allegations against him and on some of Nicole's behaviors. She had not actually disclosed sexual abuse at the time of the referral, however.

PSYCHOSOCIAL HISTORY

Information was scarce about the early years of Nicole's life. Both parents were reluctant to share information with DFS, given that they were both under investigation for abuse and neglect. What was known was that

Sarah Stoudt Briggs, LPC, RPTS, is currently the senior case manager of the Abused Children's Treatment Services (ACTS), Inova Kellar Center, Fairfax, Virginia.

Nicole was born to parents who had divorced 2 years prior to her birth. For the first year of her life, she lived with her biological mother and a 15-year-old brother. Nicole's father would visit, and on occasion he offered to babysit. Nicole's mother reported that at first he babysat for hours at a time; however, this soon grew to days at a time and then weeks. At some point the babysitting arrangement became permanent, and Nicole began living with her father. Nicole continued to live with her father until she was placed in foster care.

Nicole was removed from her father's care when police responded to a call indicating a disturbance at a shopping mall. A woman who was shopping with her daughter at the mall had an altercation with Nicole's father and called the police. When the police responded, the father became violent, and he was subsequently arrested. The father's volatile and unpredictable behavior caused the police investigators to become concerned about Nicole's safety with him; DFS was called, and Nicole was placed in foster care. It became clear that Nicole's father was suffering from an undiagnosed and unmedicated mental illness. It was also discovered that he had a significant history of impaired functioning. He refused all forms of treatment.

Nicole was not placed with her mother because of safety concerns. There were some questions about her mother's ability to ensure Nicole's safety. It appeared that she not only was aware of the bizarre behaviors of Nicole's father, but also knew that he was capable of abusive behavior. It was discovered that Nicole's father had previous charges of sexual, physical, and emotional abuse against him regarding Nicole's 15-year-old brother. These allegations were made when Nicole's brother was 4 and were almost identical to those that would soon be made about Nicole. Because Nicole's mother was living with the father during that time period and was not able to protect her son, her parental rights were terminated. It was unknown how the 15-year-old came to live with his mother again. However, these facts would not go unnoticed in Nicole's case, and DFS personnel were supervising any visits that Nicole had with either parent.

Once in foster care, Nicole began exhibiting a host of symptoms. Because many of these symptoms pointed to the possibility of trauma—specifically, sexual and physical abuse—she was referred to the ACTS program.

ISSUES SUGGESTED BY PRESENTING PROBLEMS

Nicole's symptoms were severe and impaired her functioning on all levels. Even when I think about them now, I am momentarily overwhelmed. She exhibited many of the more common symptoms associated with abuse: sexualized behaviors, aggression, hypervigilance, difficulty sleeping, nightmares, regressive behaviors, poor boundaries, hallucinations, and difficulties with toileting. In addition to these symptoms, there were others not so easily attributed to abuse. For example, she talked in what appeared to be a different language; she would call herself by other names; she was preoccupied with "powers"; and she had frequent fluctuations in mood and poor affect modulation.

It seemed extremely likely that Nicole had experienced some type of abuse, and it would be critical to understand her symptoms in the context of her father's untreated mental illness. He had been her primary caretaker, and she had learned her interpersonal skills from him. There is also some evidence that supports genetic predispositions to mental illness. Now that Nicole had been placed in foster care, there would be an opportunity to gauge her progress in her new, more stable environment.

SYSTEMIC ISSUES

From the limited information that could be gathered from Nicole's biological mother, it was apparent that Nicole had been exposed to domestic violence between her parents, which might have contributed to her mother's complacent behavior. Nicole's contact with her biological mother was inconsistent and always occurred under the watchful eye of her father. In fact, the only thing that was consistent in Nicole's life was her father. He appeared to be ever-present and possibly overprotective of his relationship with Nicole. He himself reported that he let his "baby" do whatever she wanted. He did not allow her to attend preschool or day care, and he rarely interacted (or allowed Nicole to interact) with other family members.

Nicole's foster home environment provided a stark contrast to her first 4 years of life. She lived with an African American couple, and both parents worked in a child-related field. Her foster mother was a very calm, gentle, understanding woman who provided Nicole with consistent structure, nurturance, guidance, and patience. In addition, Nicole attended day care and preschool for the first time in her life. Because of Nicole's lack of socialization, all of these changes were difficult for her and presented many challenges. Nicole's difficulties during this transition emphasized her symptoms and the extent to which they impaired her functioning. The severity of symptoms and Nicole's foster parents' incredible ability to advocate for her resulted in the establishment of a professional team committed to Nicole's stabilization. As I worked with Nicole, I exchanged a constant stream of information and feedback with her foster parents, her DFS social worker, her foster care worker, her teacher, and her day care provider.

TREATMENT PLAN

Before Nicole even walked into my office, I knew that this would be one of my most challenging cases. I had been warned about the severity of her symptoms and the instability of her father. I had already had contact with at least three other professionals assigned to the case, each of whom stressed the severity of this case and expressed their high hopes that treatment would bring some slight degree of order to the chaos that seemed inherent in Nicole's life.

My immediate priority was to help Nicole regain a sense of stability and security. Without consistent and predictable environments (i.e., home, day care, and therapy), Nicole was at risk for further deterioration. I had traditional treatment goals that I would address through the assessment and ongoing therapy. However, I would consider treatment successful if Nicole could have a safe and reparative experience. Although this is an important goal with all children, with Nicole it was essential. She was a child who had never before experienced or been exposed to a safe, consistent, or predictable environment, and the change to such an environment was probably provoking some anxiety even though it was a positive one. I was hoping that if I set the stage carefully, Nicole would be able to do the work successfully. I relied on the process of nondirective play therapy to set the necessary foundation for Nicole's treatment.

TREATMENT GOALS

My first goal with Nicole was to complete an extended developmental assessment of her functioning and make recommendations regarding future services. Specifically, I assessed her general developmental status; identified the presence of clinically significant symptoms; and determined how both sets of factors might affect her overall functioning. After the assessment was completed, I made a recommendation that she continue in individual therapy with the following two goals: stabilization of mood, and increased feelings of security. Once these two goals were complete, the focus of treatment would shift to Nicole's thoughts and feelings regarding her biological parents, the various family changes, and her (by now verified) history of abuse.

INDICATORS OF TREATMENT PROGRESS

The first and most obvious indicator of progress would be Nicole's ability to modulate her affect. Progress in this area would indicate that her world felt more manageable to her. It might also indicate that she had developed additional coping skills with which to negotiate her world. I expected that these changes would occur first at home and then in her day care and preschool environments. I also expected that her mood instability might linger throughout her therapy sessions, given the information she would be processing. I relied heavily on her foster parents, teacher, and daycare provider to monitor her progress outside the therapy office; therefore, I maintained contact with them periodically throughout treatment. The treatment team was responsive and willing to follow my directives. The case management of Nicole's treatment was intensive, but this was necessary for Nicole's progress.

The second indicator of progress would be Nicole's developing sense of what it was like to experience security. She would be able to identify safe people and places in her life, and would gain a new understanding of personal space, physical and emotional boundaries, and reciprocal respect. In addition, it would be critical for Nicole to utilize the lessons she learned in treatment outside of the therapy sessions. I would inform her caretakers about the lessons Nicole was learning in therapy and the vocabulary I was using, so that they would be able to reiterate these lessons across settings and situations.

The third indicator of progress would be Nicole's development of mastery over her feelings, particularly as they related to her biological family. Specifically, I hoped that she would be able to identify and verbalize (or show through play) her feelings about her biological parents, without being overwhelmed by her emotions and reverting to maladaptive behaviors such as regression.

The final indicator of progress would be Nicole's becoming able to function in an age-appropriate manner. She would be able to respect limits; to build friendships; to trust her caretakers; and to excel in school, both socially and academically.

TIME FRAME

The extended developmental assessment process may take as many as 12 sessions, depending on the child. I anticipated that Nicole's assessment would be quick (3–4 sessions), due to her expressive nature and the severity of her symptoms. However, this was not the case. Her symptoms were so complex and at times so bizarre that they were difficult to evaluate. In addition, because so much was unknown about her history with her biological family, it was difficult to put these symptoms into context. The assessment took 10 sessions.

After completing the assessment, I expected that Nicole would be in treatment for at least 12 months. This assumption was based on the severity of her symptoms, as well as on the continuing changes within her family. While in treatment, she endured many changes in visitation with her biological parents, ending with the termination of their parental rights. She was also adopted by her foster parents. Although I viewed this as a positive change, the preparation for adoption was also processed.

I was also very aware that Nicole might need a higher level of care than weekly outpatient therapy. In fact, at one point in her treatment, I did increase her sessions to twice a week.

PLAY TECHNIQUES

My approach to Nicole's treatment was flexible; it depended on her needs and on what she presented at the time of her sessions. I began my treatment with a nondirective approach. I surmised from the history I had received that her life had been chaotic and that she had experienced feelings of helplessness about the changes in her life. Given these two factors, I considered the probability that her problematic behaviors had arisen in an attempt for Nicole to gain a sense of control. The most effective way I could assist her with this task would be to provide her with the opportunity to explore her thoughts and feelings in her own way and at her own pace.

THERAPY SESSIONS

I felt apprehensive prior to my first session with Nicole, because she had been described by her social worker as "uncontrollable." I wondered how she would present in our first meeting. I introduced myself to Nicole, and she separated easily from her foster mother. Her apparent lack of fear or worry concerned me. It occurred to me, however, that this experience of meeting and going with strangers had been commonplace for her over the last few weeks.

Nicole's foster parents had prepared her for the sessions by saying that she was going to see a person "who has lots of toys and will help you with your feelings." They did not give Nicole any indication that this was a treatment program for children who had been sexually abused. I was therefore surprised when Nicole began to disclose sexual abuse on the way up to my office. She stated, "My daddy hurt me down there," as she pointed to her vagina. She continued by saying, "He licked me down there. He's nasty." My assessment had begun in the stairwell to my office. I wondered about the quick disclosure and considered the possibility that Nicole was being coached. It was also possible that she had overheard or been told by someone that this was a sexual abuse treatment program, and that she therefore was doing what she thought she was supposed to do. I also pondered whether her disclosure was simply due to an increased sense of safety in her environment. I responded to her immediately, believing that a swift response was more important than the possibility that someone would overhear our conversation. I told her, "I'm sorry to hear that your daddy licked you down there, and it was not OK for your daddy to touch your private parts." She seemed satisfied with my response, and she turned and continued walking to the therapy office. Once in the therapy office, I explained the rules, stressing the main point: "We can do almost anything we want in here as long as we keep each other safe." Little did I know how many times I would remind Nicole of this rule over the course of our treatment. She spent the rest of the session participating in exploratory play, looking at many of my play therapy toys, games, and props. She was immediately drawn to the sand tray, which would serve as a major tool in her therapy. She engaged me in her play by asking me to help her bury the "monsters," utilizing a witch figure. This signaled the beginning of her posttraumatic play.

When I took Nicole to meet her foster mother in the waiting room after her first therapy session, she said, "My daddy hurt me." She then asked where her father was and tried to kiss her foster mother with an open mouth and tongue. Her foster mother later explained to me that Nicole had recently begun disclosing her sexual abuse, was preoccupied with thoughts about the abuse, and was repeatedly speaking about her father.

Over the course of the next few weeks, I observed some of the behaviors that had been described by Nicole's caretakers. Although she appeared to be excited to see me, sessions would usually begin with Nicole's calling me names like "nasty girl," "crazy head," and "grossy girl." There was no anger associated with the name calling, and at times she even seemed to think the name were funny. I also noticed some of the odd behaviors that had been described to me. At times Nicole would talk in what appeared to be a different language; she would speak about "powers" and roll her eyes back in her head. She would also mimic some of my mannerisms. In addition, she exhibited difficulties with affect modulation; for example, she could go from crying to laughing hysterically in a matter of minutes. In making a diagnosis, I considered the possibilities of PTSD and a dissociative disorder. I also considered the systemic impact of her father's untreated mental illness on Nicole's first years.

In her play with the sand tray, Nicole continued to bury "monsters," stating that her father had licked her. She also made disclosures that her biological mother was involved in the abuse—an issue that remained uncertain throughout treatment. Although I did not discount the possibility of her mother's direct involvement in the abuse, it also seemed possible that Nicole generalized her abuse to include her mother because she associated her mother so closely with her father (her mother never had a visit with Nicole unless her father was present). Nicole's therapy sessions always ended with my having to set a limit about leaving. She found it very difficult to leave the office. Her behavior fluctuated between compliance and temper tantrums. Thus I introduced an ending ritual in which she could choose a sticker. This served two purposes: The choice allowed her some control at the end of the session, and the sticker served as a transitional object—something she could take from my office with her.

During the sixth session, Nicole's posttraumatic play began to exhibit greater detail. Her play had become repetitive and appeared to symbolize the dynamics of her abuse. Themes in her play included vulnerability, danger, and the need for protection. As she repeatedly exposed herself to the posttraumatic play, and as it began to change and evolve, she appeared to gain some mastery over her trauma and related feelings.

At the start of this sixth session, I asked Nicole whether she had forgotten to talk to me about something during her last session. (Her foster mother had telephoned to tell me that Nicole seemed distraught, because she had forgotten to tell me something.) She immediately responded by saying, "Mommy and Daddy licked me." She then moved quickly to the sand tray and located the witch and baby figures, labeling the witch as "bad." The witch then began "hurting" the baby. I saw this play as a sign of progress given the fact that the play occurred on top of, versus under, the sand. (Up to this point she was covering all the toys with sand). Now she was letting me witness the play. I began to ask Nicole questions about the baby: "What is the baby thinking?" and "What is the baby feeling?" Finally I asked, "Is there any way to keep the baby safe?" She immediately picked an angel figure to "protect" the baby and a "cage" (toy jail) to lock up the "scary, bad powers." She also decided that the police should be called whenever there was trouble. Her play then changed from sand play to imaginary play, in which both Nicole and I were playing the roles of police officers. She directed the play, stating that when the witch tried to hurt the baby, we should call the police. The police would then come and put the witch in jail. Nicole added that the police should "handcuff the witch when they put *him* in jail." (Interestingly, Nicole had witnessed her father being handcuffed and taken away by police the day she was placed in foster care.) She recreated this scene consistently. By the end of the session, she was speaking for all the characters in the play—including the angel, who began to say, "You can't hurt the baby."

Nicole's affect also evolved throughout the session. She gradually grew very excited about the play and began to laugh and smile. At the end of the session, she announced, "I kept the baby safe!" She appeared to feel empowered by the play; that is, she seemed to feel powerful because she could keep the baby safe. This was the first session that Nicole left the playroom without my needing to reinforce a time limit. In the waiting room, she excitedly told her foster mother about the session and was very proud of the fact that she had kept the baby safe. Nicole then turned to me and asked, "Are you going to keep me safe?" I replied that I would work with all the other people in her life to try and keep her safe. I was very careful not to make a promise, however, because it was possible that the court could decide that she would have future visits with her father. Nicole then turned to me, gave me her sticker, kissed me on the cheek, and stated, "You're my friend." Typically, when clients try to have physical contact with me or call me their friend, I view it as an opportunity to set a boundary. However, this action was such an important gesture of gratitude and trust that I stayed in the moment and accepted it as such.

The day after this session, I was interested to learn what Nicole's postsession behavior might have been, and thus I contacted Nicole's foster mother. She stated that Nicole continued to talk about the session throughout the night and the next morning. She even seemed to make a conscious connection between her play and her own situation. Nicole told her foster mother that she (Nicole) had kept the baby safe (in the session), and that since she (Nicole) was a baby, she was also safe. She took the play one step further by translating the symbolic use of the toys: "Daddy and Mommy are like the witch, and they should be locked up."

At the beginning of the next session, Nicole's foster mother reported that they'd had a great week. This was noteworthy, given the fact that temper tantrums were a daily occurrence. Once Nicole entered the playroom, she immediately asked, "Where is the witch?" I stated that the witch was where she had left him. (Prior to the session, I made sure that the witch was still in the "cage" where she'd left it after the last session.) She then located the cage and the baby, and began to recreate the scenario from the previous week. She did this twice before requesting to use the art supplies. Although she switched media, the theme of the session continued. She began to paint a picture of the "power, witch, baby, and angel." While painting, she stated, "Mommy and Daddy licked me." She then pointed to her buttocks and vagina to indicate where they licked her. She ended her painting by saying, "You keep me safe." After this, her play moved from the painting to the doctor's kit. She role-played that she was the doctor taking care of a patient (she assigned me the role of the patient). The patient was "hurt all over by the witch." When doctor's play occurs, it is significant for a variety of reasons. The most obvious reason is that it may symbolize the nurturing of a child who has been hurt. However, in this particular case it might also have been an actual reenactment of a medical exam that Nicole experienced: shortly before the beginning of treatment, she had undergone a medical exam for possible sexual abuse at a local hospital. This exam was conducted by nurses with specialized training in detecting and storing evidence of such abuse. These exams can be stressful for children who have been abused, but they may also feel reassured that they are physically healthy.

During our next session, Nicole reenacted the posttraumatic play from previous sessions. She then found a baby doll who was "disabled" (sitting in a wheelchair), and she began to role-play that she was the doctor checking on the baby. Nicole removed the baby's diaper and began using toy medical instruments to check the baby's buttocks and vagina. I asked whether there was something wrong with the baby's private parts. She replied that the witch hurt them. After repeatedly examining the baby, she went to look for and found the witch figure. She the hit the witch figure, stating, "You're bad and you hurt the baby." Nicole seemed to be expressing her anger at her abuser through her play, even though she did not directly say that. There is some controversy among sexual abuse counselors about the necessity for children to speak directly and specifically about their abuse. In this example, Nicole was using play therapy (with an established safe distance) to show her feelings of vulnerability (the hurt baby), danger (the witch), and restoration (being cared for by a doctor).

The doll that Nicole selected and utilized in this portion of the therapy became very important to her. I don't think it was coincidental that she chose the "disabled" doll for her play. This baby in the wheelchair was a concrete symbol of her emotional hurt, which she would have had difficulty expressing with the other dolls in the therapy office. (However, not every therapy office is stocked with a "disabled" doll. Other options might be to have Band-Aids or bandages accessible so that they can be applied to generic dolls.)

At another point in treatment, the doll became a useful part of an intervention for Nicole. As I have mentioned earlier, Nicole struggled with the ending of therapy sessions. In an attempt to make this transition easier and to decrease her persistent difficulty, I tried a number of techniques. I first introduced a transitional object, the sticker. Then she and I began setting an alarm clock alerting her to the last 5 minutes of the session. Lastly, I began taking pictures of her sand trays for her to take home.

Nevertheless, her behaviors escalated to the point that at the end of one particular session she began to have a tantrum and actually hit me. Her tantrum ended with her crying uncontrollably and repeating, "I'm sorry." I decided to shift to a more directive approach that might provide her with greater structure and containment. At our next session, Nicole once again played with the doll, rocking it and singing, "Baby will be OK." She seemed very involved with the play and had a concerned look on her face. The end of the session was fast approaching, so I explained that the baby might feel safer if Nicole chose a safe place for the baby where she could wait for Nicole to return. Nicole was immediately energized by this idea and picked a safe place in my office for the baby (under a chair). Upon leaving (without any limit setting), Nicole said, "Don't worry, baby. You're safe with Sarah. Mommy and Daddy won't hurt you." Amazingly, Nicole had found a way to feel safe about leaving the therapy session by leaving the doll in my care. Over the course of the next few weeks, Nicole covered her doll with a blanket, hung necklaces around her neck, and seemed to reinforce the doll's comfort level in other ways before leaving the room.

In order to understand the significance of this aspect of Nicole's play, it is important to explain that visitation with both of her parents had now been stopped, because of their inappropriate behavior during the visits and her severe behavioral regression after these visits. Nicole remained constantly worried that her parents would come and take her away, in spite of the suspension of visits. She would even report seeing her father lurking in trees and coming into her bedroom to watch her sleep. These ideas were not as paranoid as they might appear: Although her father did not know her whereabouts, he continually warned professionals that he would get his "baby" back. On one occasion, Nicole's father did locate her and tried to make contact with her at school, day care, and her bus stop. Fortunately, everyone was aware of the court order forbidding Nicole's father to have contact with her, and they refused him access. Nicole's security was a major concern to Nicole and her professional team.

For the next few months, her foster parents and I tried to instill a sense of security in Nicole. Over time, visions of her father subsided, and her play also indicated a reduction in her fear. Nicole was always very interested in bugs, and she brought a bug to one of our therapy appointments. She found it outside my office and put it in a cup until she could get it inside. Once she and it were in the playroom, she became very focused on finding it a safe place to live. This provided a great opportunity for an intervention called the "safe environment project" (Sobol & Schneider, 1996). This arts and crafts intervention consists of constructing and decorating a "safe place" for a miniature toy animal of the client's choosing. Undertaking this project allows the child to think about what is needed in an environment in order for the animal to feel safe. I suggested to Nicole that she build a safe environment for her bug.

Nicole was very excited about the idea and quickly began collecting her supplies. Her safe place had to have a door and window like her foster parents' house. She also made sure that it included food, a bed, a roof, and toys. During the building of her safe place, she began to talk to the bug, stating, "Don't worry. Mommy and Daddy won't get you." She continued to say this, and then looked at me and said, "Keep Mommy and Daddy away. If they come, you slap them." She was immersed in her play and seemed to be unaware of anything else around her. I noticed that she used a very nurturing voice with the bug and talked very calmly in a sing-song manner, similar to the way I had observed her foster mother talking to her. She went on, "Don't let Mommy and Daddy hurt the bug. She's just a little girl." I was struck by this statement. Once again, Nicole had made the connection between her play and her life—this time, between the bug's need for safety and her own. However, the best part of the session was still to come. At the end of the session, Nicole excitedly took the bug and its new home to show her foster mother, and briefly explained the reason for the elaborate creation. As Nicole was leaving, she leaned over the safe place and whispered into the bug's cup, "Don't worry, bug. You don't need to be scared any more." This was a clear indication that her own fears were decreasing.

Over the last few months of Nicole's treatment, she showed many indicators of progress: She was not struggling with expressing her emotions, and her foster parents reported that she rarely had temper tantrums any more. These reports were consistent with both the day care provider's and teacher's reports. In addition, her symptoms of PTSD (i.e., nightmares, difficulty sleeping, hypervigilance, and intrusive thoughts) and other presenting symptoms had all disappeared.

Nicole's therapy sessions were no longer permeated by themes of vulnerability, danger, and protection. However, on one last occasion near the end of treatment, she recreated the scenario of the witch's harming the baby. This time, after the police arrested the witch and put him in jail, the witch began asking the baby to let him out of jail. The baby made the witch explain why he was sorry and why he deserved to be let out of jail. The baby would then decide whether or not the witch deserved to be let out. In this expanded play, the baby had control over the witch's fate, symbolizing Nicole's ultimate struggle for control and mastery over her feelings associated with her abuse and/or abuser.

Eventually Nicole's therapy focused on more age-appropriate topics and developmental challenges, such as making friends and starting school. Nicole completed her treatment goals, and after 18 months of therapy she successfully terminated treatment and was adopted by her foster parents. It has been 2 years since she completed treatment, and her adoptive parents report that she continues to do well. She is excelling in school, is thriving at home, and has many friends.

SUMMARY

Nicole was a 4-year-old with an extensive history of physical, emotional, and sexual abuse. She endured an environment of chaos, inconsistency, and limited structure before being placed in foster care. As a result, she was struggling to function in her new environments. After a clinical assessment was completed, it was clear that Nicole would need ongoing individual therapy to enable her to gain a sense of control and mastery over her life. She participated successfully in 18 months of treatment and achieved all of her treatment goals.

The first phase of treatment consisted of creating a safe environment for Nicole, both in and out of the therapy room. This was probably the most effective part of her treatment and required the involvement and cooperation of all the instrumental people in her life. Without this foundation, she would not have been able to attempt the harder tasks of processing her feelings about her biological family and her abuse. In addition, the increased structure and consistency from caretakers assisted Nicole with mood stabilization. The more predictable her environment became, the more trust and security she developed.

The later phase of treatment focused on processing her feelings about her biological family and her abuse. She did this through nondirective play therapy, which allowed her to feel control in her therapy process and to work at her own pace. Gradually she identified her feelings while negotiating ways to cope with them. Ultimately she gained a sense of personal power and independence. At the conclusion of treatment, Nicole proved to be an extremely resilient child who had thrived in an appropriate, safe, and empathic environment.

Epilogue

This book crystallizes my thinking about helping abused and traumatized children. It has also made me realize how much I have learned from colleagues and their writings and lectures—and, even more importantly, from the children and family members whom I've met over the years and who have allowed me into their lives (sometimes reluctantly).

I don't see myself as an expert with all the answers. Instead, I see myself as an explorer who has learned to identify important guideposts as I travel, and I realize that there is always much to learn from taking unexpected turns off the path.

I rely on my intuition, my training, my experience, and what I perceive as my clients' internal resources, which they access and utilize in amazingly apt and creative ways. I believe that my greatest responsibilities are to keep trying to create a safe environment, to be patient, to hear what is not spoken out loud, to see what is not shown obviously, to decode symptomatic behaviors, and to trust that each such behavior has a helpful intent.

I turned 58 as this book went to press, and I look back and note that I have spent the past 33 years of my professional life dedicated exclusively to the prevention and treatment of child abuse. I feel proud of myself for this focus, and I am grateful to many for the generous recognition and attention I've received when I speak, write, or teach. I'm also proud of seeking more and more training; I am never content to develop rigid thinking about anything. I continue to be open to new ideas, and I will continue to integrate helpful approaches into my work as best I can.

One of my proudest achievements to date has been to obtain my art therapy credential. I worked very hard to achieve that goal, and it was one of the best personal and professional decisions I ever made. I met superb mentors, teachers, and supervisors along the way—most notably Carol Cox, Barbara Sobol, Barry Cohen, Cathy Malchiodi, and Audrey di Maria—and I am indebted to them for their wisdom, enthusiasm, and ability to communicate with great clarity and passion. I think it was Barbara Sobol who first taught me about "countertransference drawings," in which you put pen (or, preferably, chalk pastels) to paper, discharging whatever feelings and thoughts you have regarding a client or a session. This strategy is very liberating as colors, shapes, lines, images, or words fill the paper. It was a joy to learn this technique, and to this day I find it immensely useful.

This is an exciting time to be a professional in the field of child maltreatment. Talented, responsible clinicians and researchers are doing more and more impressive work—and there is much yet to learn. Never before has there been such a large group of interested professionals advancing theories and approaches in order to help abused and traumatized children. Each approach seems to have its own merits, and scientific data are increasingly guiding our preferences and amplifying our clinical choices. I am committed to continuing to observe, learn, and study so that I can best assist my clients.

References

Allan, J., & Berry, P. (1987). Sandplay. *Elementary School Guidance and Counseling*, *21*(4), 300–306.

Allred, M. T. S., & Burns, G. (1997). *STOP: Just for kids (For kids with sexual touching problems by kids with sexual touching problems)*. Brandon, VT: Safer Society Press.

American Psychiatric Association. (1980). *Diagnostic and statistical manual of mental disorders* (3rd ed.). Washington, DC: Author.

American Psychiatric Association. (20000. *diagnostic and statistical manual of mental disorders* (4th ed., text rev.). Washington, DC: Author.

Amster, F. (1982). Differential issues of play in treatment of young children. In G. L. Landreth, (Ed.), *Play therapy: Dynamics of the process of counseling with children* (pp. 33–44). Springfield, IL: Thomas.

Axline, V. (1947). *Play therapy*. Boston: Houghton Mifflin.

Bandura, A. (1977). *Social learning theory*. Englewood Cliffs, NJ: Prentice Hall.

Berliner, L., & Briere, J. (1997). Trauma, memory and clinical practice. In L. M. Williams & V. L. Banyard (Eds.), *Trauma and memory* (pp. 3–18). Thousand Oaks, CA: Sage.

Berliner, L., & Elliott, D. M. (2002). Sexual abuse of children. In J. B. E. Myers, L. Berliner, J. Briere, C. T. Hendrix, C. Jenny, & T. Reid (Eds.), *The APSAC handbook of child maltreatment* (2nd ed., pp. 55–78). Thousand Oaks, CA: Sage.

Borrego, J., Urquiza, A. J., Rasmussen, R. A., & Zebell, N. (1999). Parent–child interaction therapy with a family at high risk for physical abuse. *Child Maltreatment*, *4*(4), 331–342.

Bosquet, M. (2004). How research informs clinical work with traumatized young children. In J. D. Osofsky (Ed.), *Young children and trauma: Intervention and treatment* (pp. 301–325). New York: Guilford Press.

Boyer, L. R. (1970). *The Lowenfeld world technique*. Oxford: Pergamon Press.

235

Braun, B., & Sachs, R. (1985). The development of multiple personality disorder: Predisposing, precipitating, and perpetuating factors. In R. Kluft (Ed.), *Childhood antecedents of multiple personality* (pp. 37–64). Washington, DC: American Psychiatric Press.

Briere, J. (1996). *Trauma Symptom Checklist for Children (TSCC): Professional manual.* Odessa, FL: Psychological Assessment Resources.

Brody, V. (1978). Developmental play: A relationship focused program for children. *Journal of Child Welfare, 57*(9), 591–599.

Brody, V. (1993). *The dialogue of touch: Developmental play therapy.* Treasure Island, FL: Developmental Play Therapy Associates.

Brohl, K. (1996). *Working with traumatized children: A handbook for healing.* Washington, DC: Child Welfare League of America.

Brooke, S. L. (1995). Art therapy: An approach to working with sexual abuse survivors. *The Arts in Psychotherapy, 22,* 447–466.

Brown, M., & Brown, L. K. (1988). *Dinosaurs divorce.* Boston: Little, Brown.

Burns, G. W. (2005). *101 healing stories for kids and teens: Using metaphors in therapy.* Hoboken, NJ: Wiley.

Burns, R. C., & Kaufman, S. H. (1972). *Actions, styles and symbols in Kinetic Family Drawings (K-F-D): An interpretive manual.* New York: Brunner/Mazel.

Bühler, C. (1951). The World Test: A projective technique. *Journal of Child Psychiatry, 2,* 4–23.

Cabe, N. (2002). *Woody and Willy: A book about touching.* Royal Oak, MI: Self-Esteem Shop.

Carey, L. (1999). *Sandplay therapy with children and families.* Northvale, NJ: Aronson.

Cattanach, A. (1992). *Play therapy with abused children.* London: Kingsley.

Christophersen, E. R., & Mortweet, S. L. (2001). *Treatments that work with children: Empirically supported strategies for managing childhood problems.* Washington, DC: American Psychological Association.

Ciottone, R. A., & Madonna, J. M. (1996). *Play therapy with sexually abused children: A synergistic clinical–developmental approach.* Northvale, NJ: Aronson.

Cohen, B. M., Barnes, M., & Rankin, A. B. (1995). *Managing traumatic stress through Art: Drawing from the center.* Lutherville, MD: Sidran Press.

Cohen, B. M., & Cox, C. T. (1995). *Telling without talking: Art as a window into the world of multiple personality.* New York: Norton.

Cohen, J. A., Deblinger, E., Mannarino, A. P., & de Arellano, M. A. (2001). The importance of culture in treating abused and neglected children: An empirical review. *Child Maltreatment, 6*(2), 148–157.

Cohen, J. A., & Mannarino, A. P. (1993). A treatment model for sexually abused preschoolers. *Journal of Interpersonal Violence, 8,* 115–131.

Cohen, J. A., & Mannarino, A. P. (1996). A treatment outcome study for sexually abused children: Initial findings. *Journal of the American Academy of Child and Adolescent Psychiatry, 35,* 42–50.

Cohen, J. A., & Mannarino, A. P. (1997). A treatment study for sexually abused preschool children: Outcome during a one-year follow up. *Journal of the American Academy of Child and Adolescent Psychiatry, 36,* 1228–1235.

Cohen, J. A., & Mannarino, A. P. (1998). Interventions for sexually abused children: Initial treatment outcome findings. *Child Maltreatment, 3*, 17–26.

Cohen, J. A., & Mannarino, A. P. (2002). Addressing attributions in treating abused children. *Child Maltreatment, 7*(1), 81–84.

Cohen, J. A., Mannarino, A. P., Berliner, L., & Deblinger, E. (2000). Trauma-focused cognitive-behavioral therapy for children and adolescents: An empirical study. *Journal of Interpersonal Violence, 15*(11), 1202–1223.

Cohen-Liebman, M. S. (1999). Drawings as judiciary aids in child sexual abuse litigation. *Art Therapy: Journal of the American Art Therapy Association, 11*(4), 260–265.

Combs, G., & Freedman, J. (1990). *Symbol, story, and ceremony: Using metaphor in individual and family therapy.* New York: Norton.

Conte, J. (Ed.). (2002). *Critical issues in child sexual abuse: Historical, legal, and psychological perspectives.* Thousand Oaks, CA: Sage.

Crenshaw, D., & Mordock, J. (2005). *Understanding and treating the aggression of children: Fawns in gorilla suits.* Lanham, MD: Aronson.

Crisci, G., Lay, M., & Lowenstein, L. (1997). *Paper dolls and paper airplanes: Therapeutic exercises for sexually traumatized children.* Indianapolis, IN: Kidsrights Press.

Deblinger, E., & Heflin, A. H. (1996). *Treating sexually abused children and their nonoffending parents: A cognitive behavioral approach.* Thousand Oaks, CA: Sage.

Deblinger, E., Lippmann, J. & Steer, R. (1996). Sexually abused children suffering Posttraumatic stress symptoms: Initial treatment outcome findings. *Child Maltreatment, 1*, 310–321.

Deblinger, E., McLeer, S. V., & Henry, D. (1990). Cognitive-behavioral treatment for sexually abused children suffering posttraumatic stress: Preliminary findings. *Journal of the American Academy of Child and Adolescent Psychiatry, 29*, 747–752.

Deblinger, E., Stauffer, L. B., & Steer, R. A. (2001). Comparative efficacies of supportive and cognitive-behavioral group therapies for young children who have been sexually abused and their nonoffending mothers. *Child Maltreatment, 6*, 332–343.

Deblinger, E., Steer, R. A., & Lippmann, J. (1999). Two-year follow-up study of cognitive-behavioral therapy for sexually abused children suffering posttraumatic stress symptoms. *Child Abuse and Neglect, 23*, 1371–1378.

DeDomenico, G. S. (1988). *Sand tray world play: A comprehensive guide to the use of sand tray in psychotherapeutic and transformational settings.* Oakland, CA: 1946 Clement Rd., Oakland, CA: Author.

De Maria, R., Weeks, G., & Hof, L. (1999). *Focused genograms: Intergenerational Assessment of individuals, couples, and families.* Philadelphia: Brunner/Mazel.

Dundas, E. (1978). *Symbols come alive in the sand.* Aptos, CA: Aptos Press.

Efran, J. S., Mitchell, A. G., & Gordon, D. E. (1998, March–April). Lessons of the new genetics. *Family Therapy Networker,* pp. 27–41.

Ekstein, R. (1966). *Children of time and space, of action and impulse.* New York: Appleton Century-Crofts.

Engel, S. (1995). *The stories children tell: Making sense of the narratives of childhood.* New York: Freeman.

Esman, A. H. (1983). Psychoanalytic play therapy. In C. E. Schaefer & K. J. O'Connor (Eds.), *Handbook of play therapy* (pp. 11–20). New York: Wiley.

Finkelhor, D. (1984). *Child sexual abuse: New theory and research.* New York: Free Press.

Finkelhor, D., & Browne, A. (1985). The traumatic impact of child sexual abuse: A conceptualization. *American Journal of Orthopsychiatry, 55,* 530–541.

Foa, E. B., & Rothbaum, B. O. (1998). *Treating the trauma of rape: Cognitive-behavioral therapy for PTSD.* New York: Guilford Press.

Freud, S. (1955). Analysis of a phobia in a five-year-old boy. In J. Strachey (Ed. & Trans.), *The standard edition of the complete psychological work of Sigmund Freud* (Vol. 10, pp. 5–147). London: Hogarth Press. (Original work published 1909)

Friedrich, W. N. (1990). *Psychotherapy of sexually abused children and their families.* New York: Norton.

Friedrich, W. N. (1995). *Psychotherapy with sexually abused boys: An integrated approach.* Thousand Oaks, CA: Sage.

Friedrich, W. N. (1997). *Child Sexual Behavior Inventory (CSBI): Professional manual.* Odessa, FL: Psychological Assessment Resources.

Friedrich, W. N. (2002a). An integrated model of psychotherapy for Abused children, In J. B. E. Myers, L. Berliner, J. Briere, C. T. Hendrix, C. Jenny, & T. Reid (Eds.), *The APSAC handbook of child maltreatment* (2nd ed., pp. 141–157). Thousand Oaks, CA: Sage.

Friedrich, W. N. (2002b). *Psychological assessment of sexually abused children and their families.* Thousand Oaks, CA: Sage.

Furth, G. M. (2002). *The secret world of drawings: A Jungian approach to healing through art* (2nd ed.). Toronto: Inner City Books.

Gallo-Lopez, L. (2005). Drama therapy in the treatment of children with sexual behavior problems. In A. M. Weber & C. Haen (Eds.), *Clinical applications of drama therapy in child and adolescent treatment* (pp. 137–152). New York: Brunner-Routledge.

Gantt, L., & Tabone, C. (2003). The Formal Elements Art Therapy Scale and "Draw a Person Picking an Apple from a Tree." In C. A. Malchiodi (Ed.), *Handbook of art therapy* (pp. 420–427). New York: Guilford Press.

Garb, H. N., Wood, J. M., & Nezworski, M. T. (2000). Projective techniques and a detection of child sexual abuse. *Child Maltreatment, 5*(2), 161–168.

Gerity, L. A. (1999). *Creativity and the dissociative patient: Puppets, narrative, and art in the treatment of survivors of childhood trauma.* London: Kingsley.

Gil, E. (1985). *Systemic treatment of families who abuse.* San Francisco: Jossey-Bass.

Gil, E. (1991). *The healing power of play: Work with abused children.* New York: Guilford Press.

Gil, E. (1994). *Play in family therapy.* New York: Guilford Press.

Gil, E. (2003a). Art and play therapy with sexually abused children. In C. A. Malchiodi (Ed.), *Handbook of art therapy* (pp. 152–166). New York: Guilford Press.

Gil, E. (2003b). Family play therapy: "The bear with short nails." In C. E. Schaefer (Ed.), *Foundations of play therapy* (pp. 192–218). New York: Wiley.

Gil, E. (2003c). Play genograms. In C. F. Sori & L. L. Hecker (Eds.), *The therapist's notebook for children and adolescents: Homework, handouts, and activities for use in psychotherapy* (pp. 49–56). New York: Haworth Press.

Gil, E., & Drewes, A. (Eds.). (2005). *Cultural issues in play therapy.* New York: Guilford Press.

Gil, E., & Johnson, T. C. (1993). *Sexualized children: Assessment and treatment of sexualized children and children who molest.* Royal Oak, MI: Self-Esteem Shop.

Gil, E., & Rubin, L. (2005). Countertransference play: Informing and enhancing therapist self awareness through play. *Journal of Play Therapy, 14*(2), 87–102.

Goodwin, J. (1985). Credibility problems in multiple personality disorder patients and abused children. In R. Kluft (Ed.), *Childhood antecedents of multiple personality* (pp. 1–20). Washington, DC: American Psychiatric Press.

Green, R. J. (1994). Foreword. In E. Gil, *Play in family therapy* (pp. v–vii). New York: Guilford Press.

Greenspan, S. I. (1981). *The clinical child interview.* New York: McGraw-Hill.

Greenspan, S. I. (1997). *Developmentally based psychotherapy.* Madison, CT: International Universities Press.

Guerney, L. (1997). Filial therapy. In K. J. O'Connor & L. M. Braverman (Eds.), *Play therapy theory and practice: A comparative presentation* (pp. 131–159). New York: Wiley.

Guerney, L. (2003). Filial therapy. In C. E. Schaefer (Ed.), *Foundations of play therapy* (pp. 99–142). New York: Wiley.

Hanson, R. F., & Spratt, E. G. (2000). Reactive attachment disorder: What we know about the disorder and implications for treatment. *Child Maltreatment, 5*(2), 137–145.

Hembree-Kigin, T. L., & McNeil, C. B. (1995). *Parent–child interaction therapy.* New York: Plenum Press.

Herman, J. L. (1992). *Trauma and recovery.* New York: Basic Books.

Hug-Hellmuth, H. (1921). On the technique of child analysis. *International Journal of Psycho-Analysis, 2,* 287–305.

Hughes, J. N., & Baker, D. B. (1991). *The clinical child interview.* New York: Guilford Press.

International Society for the Study of Dissociation (ISSD) Task Force on Children and Adolescents. (2000). Guidelines for the evaluation and treatment of dissociative symptoms in children and adolescents. *Journal of Trauma and Dissociation, 3,* 109–134.

Jernberg, A. (1979). *Theraplay.* San Francisco: Jossey-Bass.

J. Gary Mitchell Film Company (Producer). (1995). *Tell 'em how you feel* [Videotape]. Sebastopol, CA: Producer. (Available from www.empowerkids.com

Johnson, S. M. (2002). *Emotionally focused couple therapy with trauma survivors: Strengthening attachment bonds.* New York: Guilford Press.

Johnson, T. C. (1992). *Let's talk about touching (2nd ed.).* [Card game]. South Pasadena, CA: Author. (Available from www.tcavjohn.com)

Justice, B., & Justice, R. (1979). *The broken taboo: Sex in the family.* New York: Human Sciences Press.

Kagan, R. (2004). *Rebuilding attachments with traumatized children: Healing from losses, violence, abuse, and neglect.* New York: Haworth Press.

Kalff, D. M. (1980). *Sandplay.* Boston: Sigo Press.

Kaplan, F. F. (2003). Art-based assessments, In C. A. Malchiodi (Ed.), *Handbook of art therapy* (pp. 25–37). New York: Guilford Press.

Kaplan, L., & Girard, J. L. (1994). *Strengthening high-risk families: A handbook for practitioners.* New York: Lexington Books.

Kelley, S. J. (1990). Parent stress response to sexual abuse and ritualistic abuse of children in day care centers. *Nursing Research, 39*(1), 25–29.

Kendall, P. C., & Braswell, L. (1993). *Cognitive–behavioral therapy for impulsive children* (2nd ed.). New York: Guilford Press.

Kendall, P. C. (1992). *Stop and think workbook* (2nd ed.). Merion Station, PA: Workbooks.

Kendall-Tackett, K. A., Williams, L., & Finkelhor, D. (1993). Impact of sexual abuse on children: A review and synthesis of recent empirical studies. *Psychological Bulletin, 113,* 164–180.

Klein, M. (1932). *The psychoanalysis of children.* London: Hogarth Press.

Klimes-Dougan, B., & Kendziora, K. T. (2000). Resilience in children. In C. E. Bailey (Ed.), *Children in therapy: Using the family as a resource* (pp. 407–428). New York: Norton.

Kluft, R. (Ed.). (1985). *Childhood antecedents of multiple personality.* Washington, DC: American Psychiatric Press.

Knell, S. M. (1993). *Cognitive-behavioral play therapy.* Northvale, NJ: Aronson.

Knell, S. M., & Ruma, C. D. (1996). Play therapy with a sexually abused child. In M. A. Reinecke, F. M. Dattilio, & A. Freeman (Eds.), *Cognitive therapy with children and adolescents: A casebook for clinical practice* (pp. 367–393). New York: Guilford Press.

Kottman, T. (1995). *Partners in play: An Adlerian approach to play therapy.* Alexandria, VA: American Counseling Association.

Kwiatkowska, H. Y. (1978). *Family therapy and evaluation through art.* Springfield, IL: Thomas.

Labovitz Boik, B., & Goodwin, E. A. (2000). *Sandplay therapy: A step-by-step manual for psychotherapists of diverse orientations.* New York: Norton.

Landreth, G. (Ed.). (1982). *Play therapy: Dynamics of the process of counseling with children.* Springfield, IL: Thomas.

Landreth, G. (1991). *Play therapy: The art of the relationship.* Muncie, IN: Accelerated Development.

Levy, D. (1939). Release therapy. *American Journal of Orthopsychiatry, 9,* 713–736.

Levy, D. (1982). Release therapy. In G. L. Landreth (Ed.), *Play therapy: Dynamics of the process of counseling with children* (pp. 92–104). Springfield, IL: Thomas.

Lowenfeld, M. (1979). *The world technique.* London: Allen & Unwin.

Lowenfeld, V., & Brittain, W. L. (1987). *Creative and mental growth* (8th ed.). New York: Macmillan.

Maddock, J. W., & Larson, N. R. (1995). *Incestuous families: An ecological approach to understanding and treatment.* New York: Norton.

Malchiodi, C. A. (1998). *Understanding children's drawings.* New York: Guilford Press.

Malchiodi, C. A. (Ed.). (2003). *Handbook of art therapy.* New York: Guilford Press.

Marvasti, J. A. (1993). Please hurt me again: Posttraumatic play therapy with an abused child. In T. Kottman & C. E. Schaefer (Eds.), *Play therapy in action: A casebook for practitioners* (pp. 485–525). Northvale, NJ: Aronson.

McCann, I. L., & Pearlman, L. A. (1990). Vicarious traumatization: A framework for understanding the psychological effects of working with victims. *Journal of Traumatic Stress, 3,* 131–149.

McGoldrick, M., & Gerson, R. (1985). *Genograms in family assessment.* New York: Norton.

McLeer, S. V., Deblinger, E., Henry, D., & Orvaschel, H. (1992). Sexually abused children at high risk for post-traumatic stress disorder. *Journal of the American Academy of Child and Adolescent Psychiatry, 31*(5), 875–879.

Mielcke, J. (2005). The Erica method of sand tray assessment. In C. E. Schaefer, J. McCormick, & A. Ohnogi (Eds.), *International handbook of play therapy: Advances in assessment, theory, research, and practice* (pp. 177–196). Lanham, MD: Aronson.

Miller, S. D., Duncan, B. L., & Hubble, M. A. (1997). *Escape from Babel: Toward a unifying language for psychotherapy practice.* New York: Norton.

Mitchell, R. R., & Friedman, H. S. (1994). *Sandplay: Past, present and future.* New York: Routledge.

Moustakas, C. (1959). *Psychotherapy with children.* New York: Harper & Row.

Nader, K. O. (1994). Countertransference in the treatment of acutely traumatized children In J.P. Wilson & J. D. Lindy (Eds.), *Countertransference in the treatment of PTSD* (pp. 179–205). New York: Guilford Press.

Nader, K. O., & Pynoos, R. S. (1991). Play and drawing: Techniques as tools for interviewing traumatized children. In C. Schaefer, K. Gitlin, & A. Sandrgund (Eds.), *Play, diagnosis, and assessment* (pp. 375–389). New York: Wiley.

Oaklander, V. (1988). *Windows to our children.* New York: Gestalt Journal Press.

Oaklander, V. (1994). Gestalt play therapy. In K. J. O'Connor & C. E. Schaefer (Eds.), *Handbook of play therapy: Vol. 2. Advances and innovations* (pp. 143–156). New York: Wiley.

O'Connor, K. J. (1983). The Color-Your-Life technique. In C. E. Schaefer & K. J. O'Connor (Eds.), *Handbook of play therapy.* New York: Wiley.

O'Connor, K. J. (1991). *The play therapy primer: An integration of theory and techniques.* New York: Wiley.

O'Connor, K. J. (1994). Ecosystemic play therapy. In K. J. O'Connor & C. E. Schaefer (Eds.), *Handbook of play therapy: Vol. 2. Advances and innovations* (pp. 61–84). New York: Wiley.

O'Connor, K. J. (1997). Ecosystemic play therapy. In K. J. O'Connor & L. M. Braverman (Eds.), *Play therapy theory and practice: A comparative presentation* (pp. 234–284). New York: Wiley.

O'Donohue, W., Fanetti, M., & Elliott, A. (1998). Trauma in children. In V. M. Follette, J. I. Ruzek, & F. R. Abueg (Eds.), *Cognitive-behavioral therapies for trauma* (pp. 355–382). New York: Guilford Press.

Osofsky, J. D. (2004a). Perspectives on work with traumatized young children: How to deal with the feelings emerging from trauma work. In J. D. Osofsky (Ed.), *Young children and trauma: Intervention and treatment* (pp. 326–338). New York: Guilford Press.

Osofsky, J. D. (Ed.). (2004b). *Young children and trauma: Intervention and treatment.* New York: Guilford Press.

Oster, G. D., & Gould, P. (1987). *Using drawings in assessment and therapy: A guide for mental health professionals.* New York: Brunner/Mazel.

Oster, G. D., & Gould Crone, P. (2004). *Using drawings in assessment and therapy* (2nd ed.). New York: Brunner-Routledge.

Oster, G. D., & Montgomery, S. (1996). *Clinical uses of drawings.* Northvale, NJ: Aronson.

Palmer, L., Farrar, A. R., Valle, M., Ghahary, N., Panell, M., & DeGraw, D. (2000). An investigation of the clinical use of the house–tree–person projective drawings in the psychological evaluation of child sexual abuse. *Child Maltreatment, 5*(2), 169–175.

Pennsylvania Coalition against Rape (Producer). (n.d.). *Three kinds of touches* [Videotape]. Enola: Producer. (Available from www.pcar.org)

Perry, B. D., Pollard, R. A., Blakeley, T. L., Baker, W. L., & Vigilante, D. (1995). Childhood trauma, the neurobiology of adaptation and "use dependent" development of the brain: How "states" become "traits." *Infant Mental Health Journal, 16*(4), 271–291.

Peterson, G. (1996). Diagnostic taxonomy: Past to future. In J. L. Silberg (Ed.), *The dissociative child: Diagnosis, treatment, and management* (pp. 3–26). Lutherville, MD: Sidran Press.

Peterson, L. W., & Hardin, M. E. (1997). *Children in distress: A guide for screening children's art.* New York: Norton.

Piaget, J. (1951). *Play, dreams, and imitation in childhood.* New York: Norton.

Prior, S. (1996). *Object relations in severe trauma: Psychotherapy with sexually abused children.* Northvale, NJ: Aronson.

Putnam, F. W. (1989). *Diagnosis and treatment of multiple personality disorder.* New York: Guilford Press.

Pynoos, R. S., & Eth, S. (1986). Witness to violence: The child interview. *Journal of the American Academy of Child Psychiatry, 25,* 306–319.

Rank, O. (1936). *Will therapy.* New York: Knopf.

Ratey, J. (2001). *A user's guide to the brain.* New York: Pantheon Books.

Reich, W. (1960). *Selected writings.* New York: Noonday Press.

Reinecke, M. A., Dattilio, F. M., & Freeman, A. (1996). In M. A. Reinecke, F. M. Dattilio, & A. Freeman (Eds.), *Cognitive therapy with children and adolescents: A casebook for clinical practice* (pp. 1–9). New York: Guilford Press.

Reisman, J. M., & Ribordy, S. (1993). *Principles of psychotherapy with children* (2nd ed.). New York: Lexington Books.

Reisman, J. M. (1971). *Toward the integration of psychotherapy.* New York: Wiley-Interscience.

Riley, S., & Malchiodi, C. A. (2003). Family art therapy. In C. A. Malchiodi (Ed.), *Handbook of art therapy* (pp. 362–374). New York: Guilford Press.

Roesler, T. A., & Grosz, C. (1993). Family therapy of extrafamilial sexual abuse. *Journal of the American Academy of Child and Adolescent Psychiatry, 32*(5), 967–970.

Rogers, A. G. (1995). *A shining affliction: A story of harm and healing in psychotherapy.* New York: Viking.

Rogers, C. (1951). *Client-centered therapy.* Boston: Houghton Mifflin.

Ross, C. (1991). Epidemiology of multiple personality disorder and dissociation. *Psychiatric Clinics of North America, 14*(3), 503–517.

Rubin, J. A. (Ed.). (1987). *Approaches to art therapy: Theory and technique.* New York: Brunner/Mazel.

Samuels, S. K., & Sikorsky, S. (1990). *Clinical evaluations of school-aged children: A structured approach to the diagnosis of child and adolescent mental disorders* (2nd ed.). Sarasota, FL: Professional Resource Press.

Saunders, B. E., Berliner, L., & Hanson, R. F. (Eds.). (2003, January 15). *Child physical and sexual abuse: Guidelines for treatment.* Charleston, SC: National Crime Victims Research and Treatment Center.

Saywitz, K., Mannarino, A. P., Berliner, L., & Cohen, J. A. (2000). Treatment for sexually abused children and adolescents. *American Psychologist, 55,* 1040–1049.

Schaefer, C. E. (Ed.). (1993). *The therapeutic powers of play.* Northvale, NJ: Aronson.

Schaefer, C. E. (1994). Play therapy for psychic trauma in children. In K. J. O'Connor & C. E. Schaefer (Eds.), *Handbook of play therapy: Vol. 2. Advances and innovations* (pp. 297–318). New York: Wiley.

Schaefer, C. E., & Carey, L. (1994). *Family play therapy.* Northvale, NJ: Aronson.

Schaefer, C. E., Gitlin, K., & Sandgrund, A. (Eds.). (1991). *Play diagnosis and assessment.* New York: Wiley.

Shapiro, A. (Producer). (1994). *Break the silence: Kids against child abuse* [Videotape]. (Available from Aims Multimedia, 7910 De Soto Avenue, Chatsworth, CA 91311-4409)

Sheinberg, M., & Fraenkel, P. (2001). *The relational trauma of incest: A family-based approach to treatment.* New York: Guilford Press.

Shelby, J. S. (1997). Rubble, disruption, and tears: Helping young survivors of natural disaster. In H. Kaduson, D. Cangelosi, & C. Schaefer (Eds.), *The playing cure* (pp. 143–170). Northvale, NJ: Aronson.

Shelby, J. S., & Felix, E. D. (2005). Posttraumatic play therapy: The need for an integrated model of directive and nondirective approaches. In L. Reddy, T. M. Files-Hall, & C. E. Schaefer (Eds.), *Empirically based play Interventions for children* (pp. 79–103). Washington, DC: American Psychological Association.

Shirar, L. (1996). *Dissociative children: Bridging the inner and outer worlds.* New York: Norton.

Siegel, D. J. (1999). *The developing mind.* New York: Guilford Press.

Silberg, J. L. (Ed.). (1996a). *The dissociative child: Diagnosis, treatment, and management.* Lutherville, MD: Sidran Press.

Silberg, J. L. (1996b). Therapeutic phases in the treatment of dissociative children. In J. L. Silberg (Ed.), *The dissociative child: Diagnosis, treatment and management* (pp. 113–134). Lutherville, MD: Sidran Press.

Silva, R. R. (Ed.). (2004). *Posttraumatic stress disorders in children and adolescents: Handbook.* New York: Norton.

Sjolund, M., & Schaefer, C. E. (1994). The Erica method of sand play diagnosis and assessment. In K. J. O'Connor & C. E. Schaefer (Eds.), *Handbook of play therapy: Vol. 2. Advances and innovations* (pp. 231–254). New York: Wiley.

Skinner, B. F. (1972). *Cumulative record: A selection of papers*. New York: Appleton-Century-Crofts.

Smith, J. S., & Nelson, R. (n.d.). *ThinKit Tool Cards*. (Available through ToolSmith Cognitive Technologies, 1780 South Bellaire, Suite 406, Denver, CO 80222)

Sobol, B., & Schneider, K. (1996). Art as an adjunctive therapy in the treatment of children who dissociate, In J. L. Silberg (Ed.), *The dissociative child: Diagnosis, treatment, and management* (pp. 191–218). Lutherville, MD: Sidran Press.

Spare, G. H. (1990). Are there any rules?: Musings of a peripatetic sand player. In K. Bradway, K. A. Signell, G. H. Spare, C. T. Stewart, L. H. Stewart, & C. Thompson, *Sandplay studies: Origins, theory, and practice* (2nd ed., pp. 195–208). Boston: Sigo Press. (Original work published 1981)

Steele, W., & Raider, M. (2001). *Structured sensory intervention for traumatized children, adolescents and parents: Strategies to alleviate trauma*. Lewiston, NY: Edwin Mellen Press.

Stern, M. B. (2002). *Child-friendly therapy: Biopsychosocial innovations for children and families*. New York: Norton.

Stien, P. T., & Kendall, J. (2004). *Psychological trauma and the developing brain: Neurologically based interventions for troubled children*. New York: Haworth Press.

Teicher, M. H. (2002). Scars that won't heal: The neurobiology of child abuse. *Scientific American*, March, 68–75. (Also available through www.sciam.com)

Teicher, M. H., Andersen, S. L., Polcari, A., Anderson, C. M., Navalta, C. P., & Kim, D. M. (2003). The neurobiological consequences of early stress and childhood maltreatment. *Neuroscience and Biobehavioral Reviews, 27*, 33–44.

Teicher, M. H., Dumont, N. L., Ito, Y., Vaituzis, C., Giedd, J. N., & Andersen, S. L. (2004). Childhood neglect is associated with reduced corpus callosum area. *Biological Psychiatry, 56*, 80–85.

Terr, L. (1983). Play therapy and psychic trauma: A preliminary report. In C. E. Schaefer & K. J. O'Connor (Eds.), *Handbook of play therapy* (pp. 308–319). New York: Wiley.

Terr, L. (1990). *Too scared to cry*. New York: Harper & Row.

Terr, L. C. (1991). Childhood traumas: An outline and overview. *American Journal of Psychiatry, 148*, 10–20.

Thompson, C. (1990). Variations on a theme by Lowenfeld: Sandplay in focus. In K. Bradway, K. A. Signell, G. H. Spare, C. T. Stewart, L. H. Stewart, & C. Thompson, *Sandplay studies: Origins, theory, and practice* (2nd ed., pp. 5–20). Boston: Sigo Press. (Original work published 1981)

Trepper, T. S., & Barrett, M. J. (Eds.). (1986). *Systemic treatment of incest: A therapeutic handbook*. New York: Brunner/Mazel.

Turner, B. A. (2005). *The handbook of sandplay therapy*. Cloverdale, CA: Temenos Press.

Ulman, E., Kramer, E., & Kwiatkowska, H. (1977). *Art therapy in the United States*. Craftsbury Common, VT: Art Therapy Publications.

van der Kolk, B. A. (Ed.). (1987). *Psychological trauma*. Washington, DC: American Psychiatric Press.

van der Kolk, B. A. (2005). Developmental trauma disorder: Towards a rational diagnosis for children with complex trauma histories. *Psychiatric Annals, 35*(5), 401–408.

Walsh, F. (1998). *Strengthening family resilience*. New York: Guilford Press.

Weber, A. M., & Haen, C. (Eds.). (2005). *Clinical applications of drama therapy in child and adolescent treatment*. New York: Brunner-Routledge.

Weinrib, E. L. (1983). *Images of the self*. Boston: Sigo Press.

Wells, H. G. (1975). *Floor games*. New York: Arno Press. (Original work published 1911)

Williams, M. L. (1996). *Cool cats, calm kids: Relaxation and stress management for young people*. San Luis Obispo, CA: Impact.

Zeanah, C. H., & Benoit, D. (1995). Clinical applications of a parent perception interview. In *Child Psychiatric Clinics of North America, 5*, 539–554.

Index